The PCOS Plan

Prevent and Reverse
Polycystic Ovary Syndrome
through Diet and Fasting

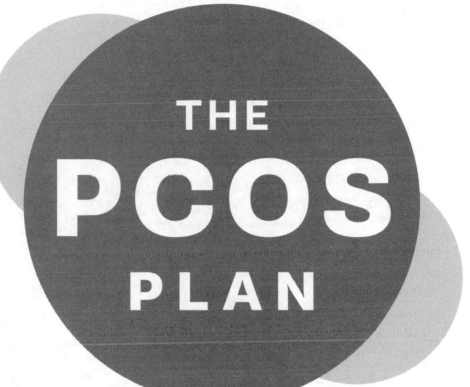

THE
PCOS
PLAN

NADIA BRITO PATEGUANA, ND
JASON FUNG, MD

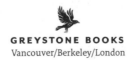

GREYSTONE BOOKS
Vancouver/Berkeley/London

Greystone Books Ltd.
greystonebooks.com

Cataloguing data available from Library and Archives Canada
ISBN 978-1-77164-460-0 (pbk.)
ISBN 978-1-77164-461-7 (epub)

Editing by Lucy Kenward
Copy editing by Rowena Rae
Proofreading by Dawn Loewen
Cover and text design by Fiona Siu
Photos on pages x and xiii courtesy of Nadia Brito Pateguana

Greystone Books thanks the Canada Council for the Arts, the British
Columbia Arts Council, the Province of British Columbia through the Book Publishing
Tax Credit, and the Government of Canada for supporting our publishing activities.

Canadä

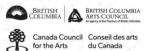

Greystone Books gratefully acknowledges the xʷməθkʷəy̓əm (Musqueam),
Sḵwx̱wú7mesh (Squamish), and səl̓ílwətaʔɬ (Tsleil-Waututh) peoples on
whose land our Vancouver head office is located.

Contents

. . . .

The Many Faces of Polycystic Ovary Syndrome

....

I HAVE A REPUTATION for getting people pregnant. In fact, people often seek me out specifically because they've heard from friends or co-workers: "Be careful. Don't go see Doctor Nadia unless you want to get pregnant." For couples living with fertility trouble, getting pregnant is a welcome miracle! I've now been a naturopathic doctor in clinical practice for more than 15 years, and my special focus is on helping women with polycystic ovary syndrome (PCOS) overcome infertility through dietary modifications.

PCOS is the most common reproductive disorder in the world. It affects an estimated 8 to 20 percent of women of reproductive age globally, depending upon the specific diagnostic criteria used.[1] Forty percent of patients diagnosed with PCOS suffer from infertility, and 90 to 95 percent of women in infertility clinics who cannot conceive due to lack of ovulation suffer from PCOS.

But my near-obsession with PCOS, fertility, and diet is not merely professional, it's also deeply personal. I became a naturopathic doctor after developing irritable bowel syndrome as a young adult.

Conventional medicine did not help, but I found some reprieve with naturopathic medicine. In 2004 I graduated from the Canadian College of Naturopathic Medicine and moved back to my home country of Mozambique, planning to work with the Ministry of Health in impoverished communities. I hoped to learn local traditional medicine to complement my naturopathic training. However, Mozambican politics are complicated and getting a job at the Ministry is not simple. I knocked on many doors, but I was repeatedly (and sometimes not so politely) turned away.

Eventually I requested a meeting with the Minister of Health himself, and after reviewing my curriculum vitae and listening to my story, he awarded me a license to practice naturopathic medicine privately. He advised me to go to Maputo, the capital of Mozambique and the city where I was born, where he said I would likely do well. I felt defeated that I couldn't follow my original plan, but with little alternative, and unwilling to turn my back on Mozambique, I did as he suggested.

I was initially worried that I had little to offer. To my surprise, though, my practice was completely full within six months. Instead of treating the poor and undernourished, I had clients who were affluent and overweight. They suffered from many of the same diseases affecting people in the Western hemisphere—the so-called "diseases of civilization," including type 2 diabetes, cardiovascular disease, cancer, and metabolic syndrome. They were suffering from "Western" diseases because their diet was modeled on the standard American diet, and their dominant concern was weight loss.

Mozambique, at the time, was considered the poorest country in the world and had some of the highest rates of malnutrition. But where rural people were starving, urban dwellers were overfed. Fast-food restaurants such as KFC and pizza joints had invaded the cities, and Coca-Cola was everywhere! From its inception, my medical practice focused almost exclusively on nutrition, diet, and weight loss.

My naturopathic training had not truly prepared me for this situation because I'd studied only a little nutrition, but as the only naturopath in Maputo, I tried my best. I created diet plans for my clients, based on my medical training and common sense. Mozambicans are a wonderful and forgiving people, and they were willing to try anything I suggested. I was very thin, and they believed what I was eating must have something to do with my low body weight.

I now realize that my diet was not particularly healthy and that my thinness might have been the result of genetics and the fact that I was a very picky and poor eater. As a child, I disliked meat and vegetables, so I snacked all day long. I lived on candy, fruit, bread, lattes loaded with sugar, and Coca-Cola. If I sat down for a meal with my family, I ate refined grains with a bit of the sauce, washed it down with a Coke, and followed that with some fruit. At night I went to bed with my bag of candies, and in the morning I started the day with a latte and toast. Only a couple of hours later, I would feel shaky and eat fruit or some more candy. I always believed that I suffered from hypoglycemia, or low blood sugar, so eating sugar every few hours seemed to make sense. Little did I know that in 30 years I would develop metabolic syndrome. Only then would I learn to eat a proper meal.

Among my first patients in this small and tightknit community in Mozambique was a South African woman named Charise who wanted to lose weight. She had a long-standing addiction to soda drinks and wanted to "detox," so I counseled her on a diet I thought might help. Several months later, Charise booked an appointment along with her husband, Johann. I usually met with Charise alone, so I was a bit apprehensive about why they were coming to see me together. When they arrived, Johann announced that they were expecting a baby! He became emotional as he explained that for the first six years of their marriage Johann and Charise had been unable to conceive. They had undergone several rounds of expensive in vitro fertilization (IVF) without success and had finally accepted that they would never welcome their own biological child into this world. Instead they had joyfully adopted a child, who was now age seven. But "miraculously," they were now expecting their first biological child. Johann was confident that my "detox diet" was the reason they were suddenly able to conceive. Over the previous three months, Charise had successfully adopted a strict diet that eliminated sugars, even the "healthy" sources like fruit and juices. Her diet encouraged protein and healthy fats such as coconut oil, avocados, eggs, butter, and olive oil. Overcome with joy, they had come to thank me.

Charise later suffered a miscarriage and lost that child. But "miraculously," she conceived for a second time and gave birth to a healthy baby boy. Johann wanted to understand the unexpected connection between this innovative diet and their newfound fertility, but I didn't have an explanation. So early in my career, I did not know myself how Charise suddenly got pregnant. I just did not understand the profound link between diet and fertility. From a practical perspective, it didn't really matter: I simply explained to patients that sometimes a bit of weight loss and a "detox" might help them bring home a little bundle of joy.

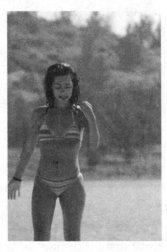

Nadia, Mozambique, 2005 (28 years old)

By age 30, I was a successful "dietician" in Mozambique. Everyone in town knew "Dr. Nadia" because I had helped many people lose weight and control their diabetes with my prescribed "Base Diet" and an occasional "detox." But I followed none of these diets myself. I kept on eating my candies and drinking my Coke. In late 2008 when my husband and I started trying to conceive, my diet was catching up with me and I started to gain weight. My lifelong acne problem was getting a bit worse. My doctor reassured me that I was thin and healthy and in good shape to have a baby, but month after month my period showed up. I would cry for days afterward and feel miserable. By the end of 2009, I realized I must be infertile. I was devastated.

By early 2010, I had gained close to 30 pounds (13.6 kilograms) but my Body Mass Index (BMI), which is a standardized measurement of weight, was still within the normal range. My acne was terrible and my hair started falling out. Blood tests showed that my androgen (male hormone) levels were high, and an ultrasound revealed numerous cysts in my ovaries. I had stopped ovulating and, therefore, could not get pregnant. I suspected I had PCOS, and my doctor confirmed it. Because I looked thin, however, my doctor overlooked all the other symptoms and simply prescribed clomiphene citrate, a type of fertility drug. I went home and just cried. All I could think about was how much I wanted a baby. I was also upset because I didn't think my doctor was doing much to help. My husband assured me that we would get through this together, and his confidence gave me the strength to take matters into my own hands.

From my professional experience, I knew fertility improved when women lost weight because I had seen so many of my clients become pregnant. My weight wasn't an issue in my lack of fertility, I thought, but I started to follow the strictest of my own diets anyway. If that's what I had to do to get pregnant, I would do it. This extremely low-carbohydrate diet, sometimes called a ketogenic diet, meant no more candies, no more Coke, no more bread.

In the first month, I lost 5.5 pounds (2.5 kilograms). Then my acne cleared up and my menstrual cycles normalized as I began to ovulate. The night before I took my next pregnancy test, I lit a candle. I was calm and positive. I asked for nothing, but I wanted a baby. In the morning, I took the test. And after 30 seconds of agony waiting for the result, the test was...positive. I was so grateful and relieved, and I immediately called my husband at work. He was ecstatic. Though he had never let on before, he admitted he had been very concerned about my physical and emotional well-being. Infertility takes a large toll on many people's work, family, and social lives. It can also drain financial resources for those people who choose to pursue IVF or other fertility treatments; I had considered IVF but it was too expensive.

While I had become pregnant, I still didn't quite understand the key role of nutrition. I threw my low-carb diet right out the window and returned to eating my candies and usual diet of small, high-carb snacks many times a day. I developed serious complications during the pregnancy, including high blood pressure and liver damage, which eventually required me to deliver the baby by cesarean section at 38 weeks. That's when my first daughter, beautiful Zinzi, came into our lives.

Unfortunately, I continued to suffer from high blood pressure and postpartum depression. One of the medications my doctor prescribed, amitriptyline, caused me to gain 20 pounds (9 kilograms) on top of the baby weight I was still carrying. Two years later, a large ovarian cyst ruptured, requiring urgent surgical removal. I was still on high blood pressure medication and having trouble sleeping. Despite my health problems, I wanted to have another baby.

When my husband and I tried to conceive a second time, the torturous journey began all over again. My doctor prescribed clomiphene once more, but by this time my BMI was in the overweight range and my health was much poorer than when I became pregnant the first time. I was eating my candies, and drinking my Coke, and taking my fertility medication. Six agonizing months later, I still was not pregnant. I remember crying constantly and feeling an overwhelming sense of doom that I would never be able to conceive again.

I stopped taking the fertility drugs and visited my friend Dr. Carolina, a Mozambican gynecologist. She told me flat out, "Of course you won't get pregnant, not even on clomiphene. You are insulin resistant!"

Until that very moment, insulin resistance related to PCOS had never crossed my mind. Much later, I realized that the low-carbohydrate diet I followed at the beginning of my first pregnancy reduces insulin, thereby improving insulin sensitivity and treating the source of my problems. But at the time, all I knew was that Dr. Carolina was right and she gave me hope. I began to take metformin, a medication to increase my insulin sensitivity—and I got pregnant the very next month.

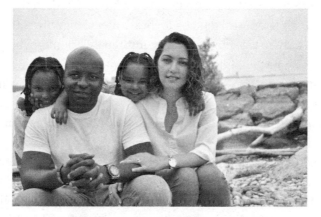

Pateguana family, July 2018, Toronto, Canada

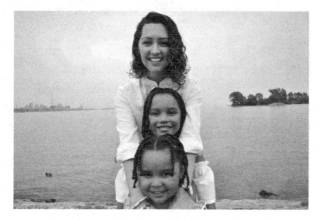

Pateguana girls, July 2018, Toronto, Canada

I experienced major complications during that pregnancy, likely because I didn't follow my low-carb diet. As soon as I gave birth to my beautiful second daughter, Zuri, I began to follow a low-carb diet again. A couple of months after she was born, I lost all my excess weight, came off all my medications, and saw my skin clear up and all my other PCOS symptoms disappear. My irritable bowel syndrome, food cravings, and mood swings also vanished. Adopting a strict low-carbohydrate diet—along with intermittent fasting—made a big difference for me. Today, over six years later, I still follow a low-carb diet along with intermittent fasting. I have not taken medication for hyperglycemia, hypertension, or depression again. I have no more symptoms of PCOS or irritable bowel syndrome. This lifestyle has been very sustainable for me, and I hope the same for you.

In 2013 my family and I returned to Canada, and three years later I met Dr. Jason Fung at a medical conference. I had followed his work for a few years on social media, and I knew that he and Megan Ramos had started the Intensive Dietary Management (IDM) program in Toronto, not far from where I was living at the time. Soon after, they invited me to bring my professional experience to their team, and I still proudly work with the IDM/Fasting Method program today. I am very fortunate to have Dr. Fung contribute his medical and scientific expertise to these pages.

Today, my passion in life is not only helping women get pregnant, but also assisting them to lose weight and take control of their health through natural dietary measures. I have learned many things about diet and fertility through my own journey and the journeys of the clients I see in my naturopathic practice, and I'd like to share that information so that you do not go through the same agony and heartbreak of infertility. Read on and good luck!

PART ONE

What Is Polycystic Ovary Syndrome?

The Diabetes of
Bearded Women

....

POLYCYSTIC OVARY SYNDROME (PCOS) has only been considered a disease in the last century, but it is actually an ancient disorder. Originally described as a gynecological curiosity, it is now the most common endocrine disorder of young women and is known to involve multiple organ systems.

EARLY DEFINITIONS

IN ANCIENT GREECE, the father of modern medicine, Hippocrates (460–377 BC), described "women whose menstruation is less than three days or is meagre, are robust, with a healthy complexion and a masculine appearance; yet they are not concerned about bearing children nor do they become pregnant."[1] This description of PCOS did not exist only in ancient Greece; it is found in ancient medical texts throughout the world.

The ancient Greek gynecologist Soranus of Ephesus (c. 98–138 AD) observed that "the majority of those [women] not menstruating are rather robust, like mannish and sterile women." The renaissance French barber, surgeon, and obstetrician Ambroise Paré (1510–1590) noted that many infertile women with irregular menses are "stout, or manly women; therefore their voice is loud and bigge, like unto a mans, and they become bearded." It's quite an accurate description from a doctor who can apparently cut your hair, cut your leg off, or deliver your children. The Italian scientist Antonio Vallisneri (1661–1730) connected these masculinizing features and the abnormal shape of the ovaries into a single disease when he described several young, married infertile peasant women whose ovaries were shiny with a white surface and the size of pigeon eggs.[2]

In 1921 French doctors Émile Charles Achard and Joseph Thiers described a syndrome that included masculinizing features (acne, balding or receding hairline, excessive facial hair) and type 2 diabetes (which used to be called adult-onset diabetes). Further cases in 1928 cemented the link between what is now called PCOS and type 2 diabetes, and these were described in the classic article "Diabetes of Bearded Women."[3] Careful observation had already revealed to these astute clinicians a syndrome that included menstrual irregularities, infertility, masculine features, and obesity with its related type 2 diabetes. The only essential feature they missed from the modern definition of PCOS was the multiple cysts in the ovary, only because they lacked the ability to carry out simple, noninvasive imaging.

DETECTION AND DESCRIPTION IN THE MODERN ERA

DRS. IRVING STEIN and Michael Leventhal ushered in the modern era of PCOS in 1935 with their description of seven women with all the modern diagnostic features: masculinization, irregular menses, and polycystic ovaries.[4] By making the connection between the lack of menstruation and the presence of enlarged ovaries, they achieved a breakthrough by merging these into a single syndrome: PCOS. The detection of enlarged cystic ovaries was difficult in the 1930s, and Stein and Leventhal achieved this either by direct surgical observation (laparotomy) or by using a now-defunct x-ray technique called pneumo-roentgenography that involved making an incision in the abdomen to introduce air and then taking x-rays. The shadow of the enlarged ovary could be seen on the film. However, in an era before effective antibiotics, this procedure was a risky one.

Dr. Stein hypothesized that some as-yet-undetermined hormonal imbalance caused the ovaries to become cystic, and he suggested that surgically removing a wedge of the ovary might help to reverse the syndrome. And indeed, this crude surgery worked. All seven women began to menstruate again and two even got pregnant. With its main features defined, interest in PCOS surged, as reflected by the large increase in PCOS articles in the medical literature.

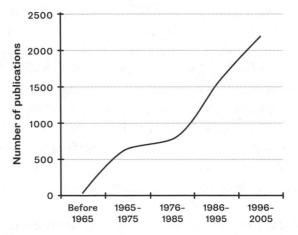

Figure 1.1. Number of publications on PCOS in the medical literature (MEDLINE)[5]

Subsequently, Drs. Stein and Leventhal performed ovarian wedge resection on another seventy-five women, restoring the menstrual cycles in 90 percent of cases and restoring fertility in 65 percent.[6] Defining the syndrome and delineating a reasonable treatment was such an accomplishment that this disease became known as Stein-Leventhal Syndrome. However, with the advent of modern medical solutions, particularly the medication clomiphene citrate, removing a wedge of the ovary is rarely done today.

Through the 1960s and 1970s, improved lab testing allowed easier detection of the typical hormonal abnormalities of PCOS. Researchers discovered that an excess of male sex hormones called *androgens*, of which testosterone is the best known, causes the masculine appearance in women. Features associated with an excess of androgens, such as acne, male-pattern baldness, and facial hair growth, are often obvious in women, but measuring these hormones is not as useful for the diagnosis of PCOS as you may think. Androgen levels in women with PCOS are only modestly elevated and vary throughout the day and throughout the menstrual cycle, so it is difficult to make a diagnosis of PCOS based on biochemical analysis alone.

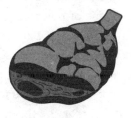 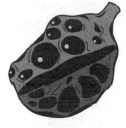

Normal ovary   **Polycystic ovary**

Figure 1.2. The normal ovary compared with the polycystic ovary. From *Polycystic Ovary Syndrome*, 2nd ed., Gabor T. Kovacs and Robert Norman, © Cambridge University Press, 2007. Reproduced with permission of the Licensor through PLSclear.

By the 1980s, the increasing availability of real-time ultrasound revolutionized the diagnosis of PCOS, because it meant laparotomy was no longer necessary to confirm the enlargement of the ovaries. In 1981 the ultrasound definition of polycystic ovaries was standardized, which allowed researchers to easily compare different cases.[7] Further refinements included the introduction of transvaginal ultrasound (an ultrasound in which the probe is inserted into the vagina), which detects ovarian cysts with more precision because the probe is closer to the ovaries. This technology soon made clear that many otherwise-normal women also had multiple cysts on their ovaries. In fact, almost a quarter of women of reproductive age had polycystic ovaries without any other symptoms. Thus, it is important to distinguish between the presence of polycystic ovaries alone and polycystic ovary syndrome.

The 1980s also saw a revolution in our understanding of the underlying cause of PCOS. The root cause of the disease was originally ascribed to excessive exposure of female fetuses to androgens, but this hypothesis was ultimately refuted. Instead, studies increasingly linked PCOS to hyperinsulinemia, literally "too much insulin in the blood," a condition commonly seen in association with insulin resistance. Because the syndrome was still known by a multitude of different names—polycystic ovaries disorder, a syndrome of polycystic ovaries, functional ovary androgenism, hyperandrogenic chronic anovulation, polycystic ovarian syndrome, ovarian dysmetabolic syndrome, sclerotic polycystic ovary syndrome, and so forth—researchers did not always know if they were talking about the same disease. To move forward in properly identifying and diagnosing the disorder, the terms would need to be standardized.

Attendees of the 1990 National Institute of Child Health and Human Development (NICHD) conference on PCOS took the first step when they agreed by consensus on the following specific criteria:
1. Evidence of excess androgens (symptomatic or biochemical)
2. Persistent rare or absent ovulatory cycles

Because these symptoms are not specific to PCOS, other diseases would still need to be ruled out. However, these so-called National Institutes of Health (NIH) criteria were a giant leap forward because proper classification allowed international collaboration between universities and researchers. Interestingly, the NIH criteria do not require evidence of polycystic ovaries, which obviously presented a problem for a disease known as polycystic ovary syndrome.

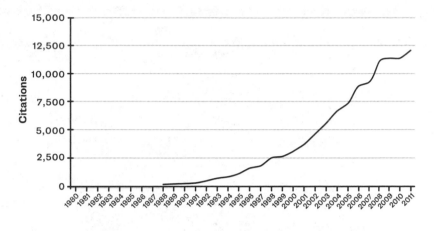

Figure 1.3. The number of scientific articles linking PCOS and insulin resistance increased from one in 1980 to about 12,000 in 2011[8]

In 2003 the second international conference on PCOS was held in Rotterdam, the Netherlands. Two new features were added to the NIH criteria. First, the mention of polycystic ovaries was introduced. It took a mere 14 years to correct that little oversight! Second, PCOS was recognized as a spectrum of disease in which not all symptoms may appear in all patients, and it was decided that a patient could be diagnosed with PCOS if they showed two of three criteria. The updated criteria, published in 2004, became known as the Rotterdam criteria:

1. Hyperandrogenism: literally, a state of too many androgens. The prefix "hyper" means "too much" and the suffix "ism" means "a state of."
2. Oligo-anovulation: literally, few or no ovulatory menstrual cycles. The prefix "oligo" means "few" and the prefix "a" means "absence of."
3. Polycystic ovaries: literally, many cysts in the ovaries. The prefix "poly" means "many."

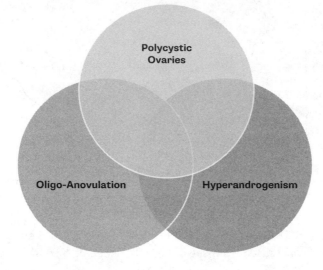

Figure 1.4. Diagnostic criteria[9]

In 2006 the Androgen Excess Society (AES) recommended that hyperandrogenism be considered the clinical and biochemical hallmark of PCOS. Without evidence of hyperandrogenism, they suggested, a person simply could not receive a diagnosis of PCOS. The AES recommendation of making hyperandrogenism a necessary criterion for PCOS diagnosis focused researchers and doctors on the underlying cause of disease rather than merely on the presence or absence of polycystic ovaries.

Today, the NIH criteria are rarely used. In 2012, an NIH Expert Panel recommended that the Rotterdam criteria be used for diagnosis. And being fairly similar to those criteria, the AES 2006 recommendations are commonly used as well.

Table 1.1. Criteria for the diagnosis of polycystic ovary syndrome[10]

NIH/NICHD[a] 1992	ESHRE/ASRM[b] (Rotterdam criteria) 2004	Androgen Excess Society 2006
Exclusion of other androgen excess or related disorders Includes all of the following: • Clinical and/or biochemical hyperandrogenism • Menstrual dysfunction	Exclusion of other androgen excess or related disorders Includes two of the following: • Clinical and/or biochemical hyperandrogenism • Oligo-ovulation or anovulation • Polycystic ovaries	Exclusion of other androgen excess or related disorders Includes all of the following: • Clinical and/or biochemical hyperandrogenism • Ovarian dysfunction and/or polycystic ovaries

[a] National Institutes of Health/National Institute of Child Health and Human Development
[b] European Society for Human Reproduction and Embryology/American Society for Reproductive Medicine

It is important to note here that although obesity, insulin resistance, and type 2 diabetes are commonly found in association with PCOS, they are not part of the diagnostic criteria.

2

The PCOS Spectrum: What PCOS Is and Is Not

....

To CONFIRM A diagnosis of polycystic ovary syndrome (PCOS), clinicians must confirm the presence of two out of the three following conditions: hyperandrogenism, menstrual irregularities, and polycystic ovaries. Because some women will present with all three criteria and others will have only two, PCOS represents a spectrum of disease. The Rotterdam criteria recognized this continuum and grouped patients into four different phenotypes:

· Frank or classic polycystic ovary PCOS (chronic anovulation, hyperandrogenism, and polycystic ovaries—3 of 3 criteria)
· Classic non-polycystic ovary PCOS (chronic anovulation, hyperandrogenism, and normal ovaries—2 of 3 criteria)
· Nonclassic ovulatory PCOS (regular menstrual cycles, hyperandrogenism, and polycystic ovaries—2 of 3 criteria)
· Nonclassic, mild PCOS (chronic anovulation, normal androgens, and polycystic ovaries—2 of 3 criteria)

The frank phenotype represents the most severe disease and is associated with metabolic diseases like obesity and type 2 diabetes and with cardiovascular risk factors like high blood pressure and cholesterol. In contrast, women with nonclassic, mild PCOS are at the lowest risk of metabolic disease.[1] Why some women with PCOS present with hyperandrogenism as opposed to anovulatory cycles is unknown.

While women may have genetic or other factors that predispose them to PCOS, lifestyle—and particularly Body Mass Index—likely determines their position on the spectrum. Weight gain moves women toward the severe end of the spectrum.[2] Weight loss, in contrast, moves women toward the less severe end of the spectrum by improving fertility, ovulatory cycles, and hirsutism.[3]

MAKING THE DIAGNOSIS

Hyperandrogenism

Male sex hormones, called androgens, are normally present in both men and women, but the normal levels for men are far higher than for women. Testosterone is the best-known androgen and contributes to many of the physical factors that distinguish men from women. It is produced in the testes in men and in the ovaries in women. Small amounts are also produced in the adrenal glands that sit above the kidneys. Testosterone helps regulate sex drive, fat distribution, and bone mass. More than 80 percent of women who present with symptoms of hyperandrogenism will eventually be diagnosed with PCOS.[4]

Common features of hyperandrogenism include
· increased facial and body hair growth (hirsutism),
· male-pattern baldness,
· acne,
· lowered tone of voice,
· menstrual irregularities, and
· clitoral enlargement (in severe cases).

The feature most commonly associated with PCOS is hirsutism, which affects an estimated 70 percent of women with PCOS. Just as with men, more testosterone increases the growth of facial and body hair in certain areas, such as the face, legs, chest, back, and buttocks.

At the same time, higher levels of testosterone can cause hair loss on the scalp, which leads to crown-pattern or male-pattern baldness. In women with hyperandrogenism, this hair gain and loss becomes very obvious.

An estimated 15 to 30 percent of PCOS patients develop acne, though it has only recently been recognized as a symptom of hyper-androgenism. Among women who complain of acne, 40 percent are eventually diagnosed with PCOS, so it is important to keep it in mind.[5] Deepening of the voice and enlargement of the clitoris indicate severe hyperandrogenism.

Serum androgen levels can be measured through blood testing. The most useful blood tests for hyperandrogenism determine levels of serum testosterone and DHEA-S (dehydroepiandrosterone sulfate), another type of androgen. These hormones fluctuate throughout the day and throughout the menstrual cycle, making it harder to define normal and abnormal ranges. Nevertheless, 75 percent of women with PCOS will have an abnormal value, if you look hard enough. Because high testosterone levels are not part of the diagnostic criteria (only clinical manifestations of it are), most clinicians do not bother to administer these blood tests.

It is worth noting that androgens also act as precursors to female sex hormones (estrogens) in both men and women. Excess adipose (fat) tissue can convert testosterone into estrogen, causing breast enlarge-ment in both men and women. This process accounts for the very obvious "man boob" phenomenon seen in some older and obese men; it is much less obvious in women. There are ethnic differences in sen-sitivities to androgens, with white people being the most sensitive and Asians being the least.

Menstrual irregularities

Dr. John Nestler from Virginia Commonwealth University estimates that "if a woman has fewer than eight menstrual periods a year on a chronic basis, she probably has a 50 to 80 percent chance of having polycystic ovary syndrome based on that single observation."[6] Irregular, absent, or rare menstrual cycles are all common symptoms of PCOS. An estimated 85 percent of women with PCOS suffer menstrual irregularities.[7] During the normal menstrual cycle, the human egg develops from the primordial follicle. It grows during the first half of the menstrual cycle and then is released into one of the fallopian tubes to be carried to the uterus, where it awaits fertilization by the sperm. Ovulation is the release of the egg from the ovary. Irregular menstrual cycles are caused by the failure of ovulation. In PCOS, the main menstrual problems are anovulation and oligo-ovulation. Anovulation means a complete lack of ovulation and oligo-ovulation refers to a lower-than-normal rate of ovulation.

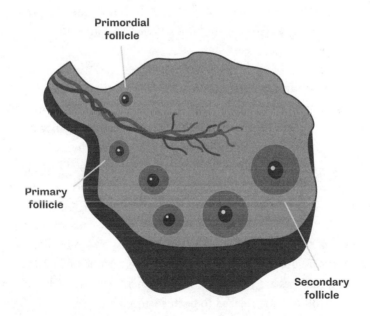

Figure 2.1. Follicle development in a normal menstrual cycle

When normal ovulation does not occur, then menstrual cycles may be completely absent (amenorrhea) or may last longer than usual (oligomenorrhea). But even having a regular cycle does not mean that ovulation has occurred normally, especially in women with other evidence of hyperandrogenism. Twenty to 50 percent of women with signs of excess testosterone and regular periods still have evidence of anovulation. This lack of ovulation will result in difficulty conceiving and infertility. PCOS is associated with recurrent miscarriages, and it is the most common cause of infertility in industrialized nations.

When I was trying to conceive, I often bought over-the-counter ovulation prediction kits that use urine strips to test for luteinizing hormone (LH). This hormone spikes just before a woman ovulates and indicates that it's baby-making time! During many of my infertile months, I noticed the same thing as many of my infertile patients do. Even when I had a menstrual cycle, whether it was regular or not (much longer than 28 days), I did not have an LH surge. In other words, I was not ovulating.

Polycystic ovaries

Follicles are collections of cells in the ovary. During a normal menstrual cycle, many follicles begin to develop and one eventually becomes the human egg that is released into the uterus at the time of ovulation. The other follicles usually shrivel up and are reabsorbed into the body. When these follicles fail to shrivel up, they become cystic and show up on an ultrasound as ovarian cysts.

The Rotterdam criteria define polycystic ovaries as being the presence of 12 or more follicles measuring 2 to 9 mm in diameter in each ovary. Two main factors influence the number of cysts. Small (2–5 mm) follicles are related to the serum androgen level and larger (6–9 mm) follicles are related to both serum testosterone and fasting insulin levels. Because 20 to 30 percent of otherwise normal women may have multiple cysts on their ovaries, the mere presence of cysts is not enough to make the diagnosis of PCOS. And there is no correlation between the number of cysts and the severity of PCOS.

WHEN WHAT LOOKS LIKE PCOS IS NOT

DESPITE THE REASONABLY clear diagnostic criteria for PCOS, certain populations present with symptoms that fit the Rotterdam criteria but do not necessarily indicate PCOS. Certain conditions, too, can look a lot like PCOS but have completely different causes and associated treatments.

Misdiagnosis in adolescents

Making the diagnosis of PCOS in adolescents is particularly tricky because irregular cycles, hyperandrogenism, and polycystic ovaries can all be found during normal puberty.

When girls first begin to menstruate (called menarche), their cycles are commonly irregular and may not always be accompanied by ovulation. In the United States, the median age of menarche is 12.4 years. The period of irregular cycles often lasts for two years or more, and the cycle intervals typically range from 21 to 45 days (average of 32.2 days). This average is quite close to the 35-day cycle that is defined as oligomenorrhea, or infrequent menstrual cycles in women of childbearing age.

Normal puberty and the irregular cycles seen in PCOS overlap significantly. To avoid overtreatment and unnecessary worry, clinicians should generally wait until the third year after menarche to confirm a diagnosis of PCOS in teens. By that time, 60 to 80 percent of girls have cycles that are 21 to 34 days long, which is typical of a normal adult cycle.

Blood testing of androgens in adolescents does not distinguish unusually high levels, because normal levels are not well defined in this age group. During puberty, there is a normal physiological increase in testosterone levels that peaks a few years after menarche. This increased testosterone leads, for example, to the familiar problem of acne during teenage years that improves or disappears in later adult years. The presence and the severity of this temporary increase in acne do not predict a later diagnosis of PCOS.

Polycystic ovaries, too, are difficult to diagnose during adolescence. In adult women, a transvaginal ultrasound, in which the ultrasound probe is inserted into the vagina, provides the clearest images of the ovary. However, this technique is usually avoided in adolescent girls, which makes the radiological diagnosis more difficult. In studies where ultrasounds were performed, 26 to 54 percent of asymptomatic adolescent girls had polycystic ovaries by imaging.[8]

Special care must be taken in labeling a patient with PCOS during their teen years, and it is often prudent to wait until after adolescence to make the diagnosis since it is not an urgent condition. If there is evidence of obesity or type 2 diabetes, these associated conditions should be treated earlier. Obesity is known to be associated with increased insulin levels, and this effect is magnified during early puberty. Fasting insulin is more than three times higher in the obese group. This effect is also seen during late puberty and adulthood, but not with such a marked difference. Testosterone levels are also likely to be higher in overweight adolescents. For example, in one study, 93.8 percent of obese preteens were found to have elevated testosterone levels versus 0 percent of the non-obese group.[9]

Differential diagnoses

Hyperandrogenism and polycystic ovaries are not exclusive to PCOS, so other diseases that mimic PCOS must be excluded by history or by physical or laboratory examination before the diagnosis can be confirmed. While most of these conditions are rare, they may be serious and require entirely different treatments, which makes the distinction important. The list of similar conditions includes

- pregnancy,
- hyperprolactinemia (prolactin excess),
- thyroid disorders,
- nonclassic congenital adrenal hyperplasia (NCAH),
- Cushing's Syndrome, and
- hyperandrogenemia (androgen excess, tumor/drug-induced)
  Let us consider some of these other conditions.

» Pregnancy

Pregnancy is by far the most common cause of menstrual irregularity. Obviously, a simple pregnancy test, either a home test or laboratory confirmation, is mandatory before confirming the diagnosis of PCOS. It would be very embarrassing to miss this simple diagnosis.

» Hyperprolactinemia

Prolactin is a hormone normally secreted by the pituitary gland in the brain that enables mammals, including humans, to produce milk. Prolactin levels normally increase toward the end of pregnancy for proper breast development in preparation for breastfeeding. Excessive prolactin in the blood when a woman is not pregnant is known as hyperprolactinemia.

A wide range of conditions may lead to hyperprolactinemia, including chronic kidney or liver disease, drug use, and thyroid disease. Another common cause is a small tumor (microadenoma) of the pituitary gland, which may oversecrete prolactin into the blood. The diagnosis of hyperprolactinemia is made by measuring the blood level of prolactin.

High prolactin levels may mimic PCOS by inhibiting estrogen and causing menstrual irregularities and difficulty with ovulation. Symptoms that may help differentiate the disease include breast enlargement and abnormal milk production.

» Thyroid disorders

The thyroid is a small gland at the front of the neck. It secretes thyroid hormone, which controls many aspects of metabolism. Too little thyroid in the body may cause weight gain, menstrual irregularities, infertility, and hair loss that may be confused with PCOS. The diagnosis of thyroid disorders is made by measuring the blood levels of the thyroid hormones (TSH, T3, T4) to rule out this easily treated condition.

» Nonclassic congenital adrenal hyperplasia

Androgens are normally produced in both the ovaries and the surface (cortex) of the adrenal glands. In rare situations, the adrenal glands overproduce androgens, resulting in a syndrome called nonclassic congenital adrenal hyperplasia (NCAH), which is reminiscent of PCOS, with irregular menstruation, hirsutism, and acne. It is a rare genetic disorder that can affect young girls and women, and there is no commonly used diagnostic test for it.

» Cushing's Syndrome

Prolonged exposure to high levels of the hormone cortisol causes Cushing's Syndrome. In some cases, tumors oversecrete cortisol. In other cases, this syndrome can be caused by synthetic cortisol (prednisone), which is used to treat autoimmune diseases (asthma, lupus) and to suppress the immune system during organ transplants. Elevated cortisol levels can cause weight gain, menstrual irregularities, and infertility, which may be confused with PCOS. While prolonged periods of stress or athletic overtraining may increase cortisol, these circumstances almost never do so to the degree that's necessary to develop Cushing's Syndrome.

Cushing's Syndrome presents with some characteristic symptoms that can help to distinguish it from PCOS. These include a pocket of fat that develops below the nape of the neck (a buffalo hump), stretch marks (striae), thinning skin, muscle weakness and atrophy, sensitivity to infections, decreases in bone density, and severe psychiatric and cognitive dysfunction. The diagnosis of high cortisol levels is made by taking a small blood sample.

» Hyperandrogenemia

Tumors in the adrenal glands or ovaries may oversecrete androgens causing hirsutism, clitoral enlargement, deepening of the voice, and male-pattern baldness. These tumors are extremely rare but potentially life-threatening. The average age of diagnosis is 23.4 years, which overlaps significantly with the age range for PCOS. Tumors typically produce far higher levels of androgen than are found in PCOS, leading to far more severe symptoms. The diagnosis of these tumors is usually made by looking at an image from a computerized tomography (CT) scan of the abdomen.

Drug-induced androgen excess is usually associated with those surreptitiously taking testosterone, mostly to enhance athletic performance. Because patients may not always admit to the use of these drugs, a high index of suspicion is necessary to make the diagnosis.

When I was diagnosed with PCOS, I checked the boxes for all three of the diagnostic criteria, even though only two out of three are necessary for the diagnosis. I had frank PCOS, the most severe phenotype, and I was devastated by this news. Today, I know there is a natural way to reverse even the worst PCOS. By understanding the underlying root cause of the syndrome, we can treat it rationally and successfully.

3

Who Gets PCOS?

....

T HE PREVALENCE OF PCOS, using the NIH criteria, ranges from 6 to 9 percent, with a strikingly similar rate globally.[1] Using the Rotterdam criteria, that rate is about 15 to 20 percent of women. This makes PCOS the most common endocrine (hormonal) disorder of young women by far. Approximately one in 15 women in the United States are affected, with similar proportions in Spain, Greece, and the United Kingdom. An estimated 105 million women of childbearing age are afflicted worldwide.

GENETICS AND PCOS
....

TO TRY TO understand why some people develop PCOS and others don't, researchers usually begin by looking for genetic influences. A large Dutch study comparing sets of identical twins with sets of fraternal twins found that approximately 70 percent of PCOS may be attributed to genetic influences.[2] A U.S. study found that sisters of patients diagnosed with PCOS are more likely to have symptoms, with an estimated 22 percent also fulfilling the full diagnostic criteria.[3] A further 24 percent of sisters had hyperandrogenism but regular menstrual cycles, likely indicating that they too had mild PCOS. In a separate study, mothers of patients with PCOS had higher androgen levels, insulin resistance, and metabolic syndrome.[4] First-degree relatives, male or female, are more likely to have evidence of insulin resistance. Despite these strong genetic tendencies, no single gene has been identified as the causative factor. This indicates that PCOS is a complex genetic disorder with multiple genes contributing small degrees of risk.

HEALTH RISKS ASSOCIATED WITH PCOS

IF PCOS WERE just about acne and a few missing periods, then it would not be so bad. Unfortunately, PCOS is associated with many health concerns, reproductive as well as general.[5] The reproductive issues include
- anovulatory cycles,
- infertility,
- disorders of pregnancy, and
- fetal concerns.

Other significant health concerns include
- cardiovascular disease,
- non-alcoholic fatty liver disease (NAFLD),
- sleep apnea,
- anxiety and depression,
- cancer,
- type 2 diabetes, and
- metabolic syndrome.

These are some of the deadliest conditions in the world, including the top two causes of death in America, cardiovascular disease and cancer. PCOS is not merely a nuisance; it is an important warning of risk. For this reason, it's worth taking a look at each of these conditions in more detail to try to understand their link with PCOS.

Reproductive concerns

» Anovulatory cycles

Most women with PCOS suffer from infrequent or absent menstrual periods, mostly caused by anovulatory cycles (ovulation is missed). PCOS accounts for 80 percent of cases of anovulation leading to infertility.[6]

» Infertility

If you do not ovulate, you can't conceive: no egg, no baby. Anovulatory cycles account for approximately 30 percent of visits to an infertility clinic, mostly due to PCOS. The Australian Longitudinal Study on Women's Health, a community-based survey of young women, found that a heartbreaking 72 percent of women with PCOS considered themselves infertile, compared with only 15 percent without PCOS. However, women with PCOS usually have difficulty conceiving rather than being completely infertile. The use of fertility hormones in the PCOS group was almost double that of the non-PCOS group. That is, the 5.8 percent of women identified as having PCOS constituted a whopping 40 percent of those seeking fertility treatments. Obviously, PCOS contributes heavily to overall use of costly fertility treatment.[7]

The financial costs of infertility are depressing. Costs in the United States range from relatively inexpensive hormonal treatments (approximately US$50 per treatment cycle) to very expensive in vitro fertilization (IVF), which in 2005 was estimated to cost upward of US$6000 to $10,000 per round of treatment. With millions of women suffering from PCOS, the total cost for infertility treatment alone in the United States is an estimated US$533 million.[8]

The possibility of being unable to conceive a child can cause severe anxiety. Celebrity chef Jamie Oliver and his wife, Jools, have spoken openly about their struggle with PCOS. They now have five children. Jools went through many rounds of hormonal treatments, and even one round of IVF, but at least two of their children were conceived spontaneously. Fertility medications such as clomiphene have been relatively successful at inducing ovulation. However, these treatments often have serious side effects—physical, psychological, and financial. While clomiphene may help women get pregnant, the PCOS-related reproductive problems don't stop there.

» Disorders of pregnancy

Losing a pregnancy can be absolutely devastating, especially if it was difficult to conceive in the first place. Spontaneous abortions occur in an estimated one-third of women with PCOS. Studies suggest that PCOS is associated with up to twice the rate of miscarriage.[9]

Rates of all pregnancy-related complications are increased among women with PCOS. Gestational diabetes, pregnancy-induced hypertension, and pre-eclampsia risks are approximately tripled. Risk of preterm birth is increased by an estimated 75 percent when compared with women in general or women who have overcome PCOS.[10] Women with PCOS are more likely to deliver by cesarean section, which itself comes with complications.

Fertility treatments may double the risk of multiple pregnancies, with all their attendant complications. Pregnancy with twins, for example, has up to 10 times the risk of the babies being small for gestational age at birth and six times the risk of delivering prematurely.[11]

» Fetal concerns

Babies of mothers with PCOS may be large for their gestational age, since hyperinsulinemia (excess insulin in the blood) is associated with increased nutrient availability. Both small and large gestational age at birth are associated with admissions to the neonatal intensive care unit (NICU), stillbirths, and perinatal mortality (infant death in the first week after birth)[12] as well as metabolic complications (type 2 diabetes, obesity, and hypertension) later in life.[13] Hyperinsulinemia in utero may affect the child's intellectual and psychomotor development too.[14]

Associated health conditions

» Cardiovascular disease

Some studies estimate that women with PCOS may have seven times the risk of developing cardiovascular disease over women without PCOS.[15] Large epidemiological studies like the Nurses' Health Study, which comprised 82,439 women, found a correlation between irregular menses (as a proxy for possible PCOS) and a higher risk of heart disease during 14 years of follow-up.[16] Although one study showed no risk,[17] a 2010 consensus statement by the Androgen Excess and Polycystic Ovary Syndrome Society estimated the increased risk at 70 to 95 percent.[18]

PCOS is a marker of greater cardiovascular risk. The association with type 2 diabetes, obesity, and cholesterol problems accounts for much of the heightened risk. Insulin resistance develops in 40 percent of women with PCOS[19] and typically gets worse with age. Women with PCOS also tend to have poor cholesterol panels. Since cardiovascular disease is already the leading cause of death in older women, this effect is especially concerning.

» Non-alcoholic fatty liver disease

The most common form of liver disease in the world, non-alcoholic fatty liver disease (NAFLD) affects an estimated 30 percent of the general population. The liver is an organ that should not normally store fat: fat should be stored in fat cells. Excessive alcohol consumption is a common cause of fat accumulation in the liver, but this can also happen in people who drink minimal alcohol. For many years, one of the leading causes of liver failure (cirrhosis) was termed "cryptogenic," which means "from unknown cause."[20] Now we know that cryptogenic cirrhosis was largely due to undiagnosed fatty liver disease. Patients with NAFLD have an estimated 2.6 times the risk of death compared with the general population, and the disease is intimately linked to type 2 diabetes and metabolic syndrome.

The first case linking PCOS and NAFLD was reported in the medical literature in 2005.[21] A 24-year-old woman diagnosed with PCOS but otherwise healthy was investigated because her bloodwork showed evidence of liver damage. A long needle was inserted into her liver and a biopsy taken. Under the microscope, to everybody's surprise, the pathology showed severe fatty infiltration.

Since then, many other studies have confirmed the tight correlation between the two diseases. Women with PCOS have two and-a-half times the prevalence of NAFLD compared with women without PCOS.[22] Approximately 30 percent of women with PCOS have evidence of liver damage by blood tests. In women of reproductive age investigated for NAFLD, 71 percent also had PCOS. Like PCOS, the occurrence of NAFLD is highly associated with metabolic syndrome.[23]

NAFLD is often underdiagnosed because there are virtually no symptoms of the disease. It is really only through blood tests that the condition is discovered. Thus, it is important to screen for this condition.

» Sleep apnea

Obstructive sleep apnea (OSA) is a condition in which the upper airway collapses during sleep. Patients cannot breathe for an instant, which causes them to wake up momentarily, though they usually don't remember. Regular sleep patterns are disrupted and sleep architecture is fragmented. The main symptoms of this disease include snoring and excessive daytime sleepiness.

The rate of OSA in women with PCOS is an astounding five to 30 times higher than in women without PCOS.[24] Like PCOS, the occurrence of OSA is highly linked to metabolic syndrome.

» Anxiety and depression

Both anxiety and depression are common among patients with PCOS, and a high index of suspicion should be maintained. Abnormal male-pattern hair growth, acne, obesity, and menstrual irregularities destroy self-esteem, especially during adolescence. Depression, anxiety, and other psychological abnormalities are more prevalent among younger women with PCOS.[25] Depression is also common among women suffering from infertility as well as chronic illnesses associated with PCOS (type 2 diabetes, cardiovascular disease, and cancer).[26]

Weight loss and lifestyle changes may improve the symptoms of PCOS as well as feelings of depression and anxiety.[27] Clinicians should regularly assess for psychological well-being.

» Cancer

Women with PCOS are three times more likely to develop endometrial cancer and two to three times more likely to develop ovarian cancer when compared with the general population.[28] Since there is a significant overlap between PCOS and obesity/hyperinsulinemia, it is no surprise that women with PCOS are also at higher risk of obesity-related cancers (such as breast cancer and colorectal cancer), which now make up 40 percent of all cancers as classified by the World Health Organization.[29]

» Diabetes

Perhaps the disease most closely associated with PCOS is type 2 diabetes, a disease of excessive insulin resistance, a trait shared by PCOS patients as well. An estimated 82 percent of women with type 2 diabetes have multiple cysts on their ovaries, and 26.7 percent fulfill the diagnostic criteria for PCOS.[30] Women with PCOS have three times the risk of developing type 2 diabetes by menopause when compared with the general population. I was one of these women. A glucose tolerance test confirmed that I had developed type 2 diabetes.

Among women with PCOS, 23 to 35 percent will have prediabetes and 4 to 10 percent will have type 2 diabetes.[31] This rate of prediabetes is three times higher than in women without PCOS. The rate of undiagnosed type 2 diabetes is 7.5- to 10-fold higher. As in the general population, the rate of type 2 diabetes among women with PCOS rises with increasing Body Mass Index. PCOS is recognized by the American Diabetes Association as a risk factor for diabetes.

Women with PCOS, particularly if obese, have a higher incidence of gestational diabetes and insulin resistance, a rate estimated to be about twice that of otherwise healthy women.[32] Gestational diabetes increases the risk of miscarriage and delivering by cesarean section or induced birth, due to the increased size of the fetus.[33] Developing diabetes during pregnancy increases a woman's risk of developing type 2 diabetes, cardiovascular disease, and metabolic syndrome in the future. Maternal obesity also increases the baby's risk of developing childhood obesity and PCOS.

Women with type 1 diabetes who are being treated with insulin are also at risk of PCOS, with an estimated 18.8 percent[34] to 40.5 percent[35] affected, compared with only 2.6 percent in the control group. PCOS is six to 15 times more common among women with type 1 diabetes, probably due to the frequent high dosage of insulin.

Women with PCOS should be screened for type 2 diabetes using an oral glucose tolerance test every three to five years. Measuring fasting glucose alone may miss the diagnosis of up to 80 percent of prediabetic patients and 50 percent of diabetic patients. If cardiovascular risk factors exist, the screening should be done annually so the disease can be diagnosed at an early stage when lifestyle measures such as dietary changes can prevent damage to the body's major organs.

» **Metabolic syndrome**

In 1988, Dr. Gerald Reaven of Stanford University termed syndrome X as a group of conditions with an unknown common factor, "X." These conditions included central obesity, high blood pressure, high triglycerides, and high blood glucose. Reaven and Dr. Ami Laws (also of Stanford University) published the book *Insulin Resistance: The Metabolic Syndrome X*[36] linking insulin resistance to metabolic syndrome and calling it the common factor in all these seemingly separate conditions.

In 2002, a National Institutes of Health report[37] defined a patient as having metabolic syndrome if three of the following five conditions are present:

· Abdominal obesity: over 40 inches (102 centimeters) for men; over 35 inches (89 centimeters) for women
· High blood glucose: over 100 milligrams/deciliter (mg/dL), or taking medication

- High triglycerides: over 150 mg/dL, or taking medication
- Low high-density lipoprotein (HDL): below 40 mg/dL for men, below 50 mg/dL for women, or taking medication
- High blood pressure: over 130 mmHg for the systolic (top) number, over 85 mmHg for the diastolic (bottom) number, or taking medication

General obesity, albeit commonly associated, is not one of the criteria. Approximately 25 percent of metabolic syndrome patients are non-obese individuals. Interestingly, high low-density lipoprotein (LDL or "bad" cholesterol) is also not a criterion, even though many doctors and professional guidelines obsess about LDL and statins.

The prevalence of metabolic syndrome in the adult American population is now estimated at 88 percent[38]—leaving only 12 percent as metabolically healthy—and this comes with an increased risk of cardiovascular disease, stroke, cancer, NAFLD, obstructive sleep apnea, and PCOS.

The link between metabolic syndrome and insulin resistance makes it a reversible dietary condition, not a chronic progressive disease.

UNDERSTANDING THE LINK BETWEEN PCOS AND ITS ASSOCIATED RISKS

PCOS MUST BE considered more than merely a disorder of excess facial hair, acne, and abnormal reproduction. Patients with PCOS have double the chance of being hospitalized compared with those without the disease. The United States spent an estimated $4 billion in 2004 on health care related to treating PCOS[39]—an amount equal to the entire gross domestic product of Barbados. Much of this cost (40.4 percent) is due to the associated type 2 diabetes.[40]

Even more sobering, this number likely underestimates the true costs, because it takes into account only the reproductive years and not the associated health risks such as type 2 diabetes, heart attacks, strokes, and cancer that may arise in the future. These diseases typically occur in a woman's post-menopausal years and are many, many times more expensive than simply treating PCOS.

Furthermore, PCOS is one of the main causes of infertility, which often leads to women seeking in vitro fertilization (a multi-billion-dollar industry). As we've seen, women with PCOS who do become pregnant are at increased risk of obstetrical complications such as gestational diabetes, pregnancy-induced hypertension (high blood pressure), and pre-eclampsia.

Though they are not part of the formal definition of PCOS, obesity leading to metabolic syndrome and insulin resistance leading to type 2 diabetes have been frequently noted in patients and affect an estimated 50 to 70 percent of women with PCOS. The close link to obesity and type 2 diabetes suggests that all three conditions have the same underlying root cause. All three are now understood as metabolic diseases, putting women with PCOS at high risk later in life for cardiovascular disease, strokes, and cancer.

Perhaps the most important associated disease is a history of weight gain that often precedes the diagnosis of PCOS. Of the obese women referred to one clinic, 28.3 percent were diagnosed with PCOS.[41] PCOS can be more common as severity of the obesity increases, but more importantly, weight loss has also been proven to reduce testosterone, improve insulin resistance, and decrease hirsutism (more on this later).

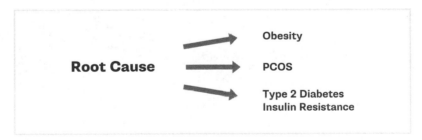

Figure 3.1. The three metabolic diseases have a root cause

PCOS, obesity, and type 2 diabetes are variable manifestations of the same underlying problem. But what is that problem? To start answering this question, we need to know what causes obesity. Once we figure that out, we can gain a clue as to the root cause of PCOS.

GABRIELLA

Gabi's story is a simple, clear-cut case of PCOS, but there's always a twist. In early 2016, Gabi decided to start a family. She had been dating Hugo for many years, and now they were going to marry. She stopped taking the birth control pill, which she had used consistently since age 18.

Once off the pill, Gabi did not have a period for many months. For the first time in her life, she developed acne, and she also gained 8 pounds (4 kilograms). Gabi saw her doctor for a check-up, expressing her concerns. Besides her weight gain, she had headaches that lasted for days and that she could manage only by taking painkillers constantly. Her bloodwork showed increased androgen (male hormone) levels, which explained the acne and missed periods. An internal ultrasound confirmed multiple small ovarian follicles and the diagnosis of PCOS. Her doctor informed her it would be difficult to get pregnant, though not impossible. She felt devastated and discouraged.

At this point, Gabi asked for my help. She had been my patient and friend in Mozambique since 2009, and she knew I'd experienced the same situation. Like me, Gabi was a young, thin woman with PCOS. At 138 pounds (62 kilograms) and 5 feet 6 inches (1.7 meters) tall, she had a BMI of 23, which was perfectly normal. I reassured her that PCOS is a reversible condition related to hyperinsulinemia and insulin resistance and that the treatment was changing her diet. We discussed the diet of low-carbs and high healthy fats, which she knew from South Africa as the Banting Diet. She started immediately.

The next month her menstrual cycle went from 73 to 56 days. Considering that a normal menstrual cycle comes every 25-30 days, she had improved tremendously, but there was still work to be done. In just one month, her headaches were nearly gone, she stopped taking painkillers, and her skin cleared up. After two months on the new diet, Gabi felt less bloated, finally lost some weight, and started to ovulate. She continued on the low-carb diet and stopped snacking completely, even on "low-carb-friendly" foods. She also began some 24-hour intermittent fasting.

By January 2017, just over four months into her new way of eating, Gabi's menstrual cycle had almost completely reverted to normal. Almost. She was late by a couple of weeks. Out of curiosity, she did a urine pregnancy test, which came out *positive*. She did a blood test right away. In Mozambique, doing a blood test is as easy as driving to the lab, ordering the test, and paying for it. This test, which is meant to be more accurate than the urine test, came back *negative*. She was devastated.

But something was not right. Her breasts were swollen and she had serious back and muscle cramps. Two other urine pregnancy tests were positive. We were worried. Could it be an ectopic pregnancy? Did she have a miscarriage? The very next day, she was able to get an appointment in nearby South Africa with her sister's gynecologist. That blood test and an internal ultrasound confirmed she was five weeks pregnant and all was well! Low-carb works. Insulin resistance is reversible.

I encouraged Gabi to stick with her low-carbohydrate diet during pregnancy to prevent gestational diabetes, knowing that women with PCOS are more prone to this and other gestational conditions. She and the baby remained healthy and well throughout the pregnancy, and Beautiful Banting Baby was born in October 2017.

PART TWO

PCOS and the Role of Hormones

What We
Know about Obesity

....

T HE WORLD HEALTH Organization defines obesity as a state of "abnormal or excessive fat accumulation." Today, it is a worldwide epidemic affecting all ages, genders, and ethnicities, and it's worsening with each successive generation. My 93-year-old grandmother never met an obese person until recently. She knew of no overweight kids in her school, family, or social circles. My 60-year-old mother had almost no overweight classmates. When I went to school, I had a few overweight classmates. They weren't unusual, but they weren't common either. My children, however, have many overweight and even obese little buddies.

Worldwide, obesity has nearly tripled since 1975. By absolute numbers, the United States is the most obese country in the world, followed closely by China and India. By proportion of population, 50.8 percent of the Cook Islands in Oceania is obese, followed by Qatar at 42.3 percent and the United States at 33.7 percent, according to a 2017 report of obesity rates by country.[1]

Obesity is commonly classified by the Body Mass Index (BMI), which compares weight to height but ignores factors such as muscle mass, age, and fat distribution. This definition limits the BMI's overall accuracy, but it is generally a simple and useful measure.

What's Your BMI?

$$BMI = \frac{\text{Weight in kg}}{(\text{Height in m})^2}$$

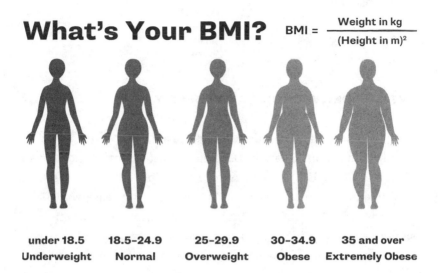

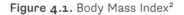

under 18.5	18.5–24.9	25–29.9	30–34.9	35 and over
Underweight	**Normal**	**Overweight**	**Obese**	**Extremely Obese**

Figure 4.1. Body Mass Index[2]

Ironically, the overriding concern of the 1970s was global hunger and the difficulty of increasing food production to avoid mass worldwide starvation. Yet, today we live with a global obesity epidemic that kills more people than does starvation. This slow-motion surge toward rampant obesity was completely unforeseen and has shocked most public health authorities. The resulting health consequences are dire. Having a BMI in the obese or extremely obese range is a risk factor for many serious health ailments, including PCOS, as well as the following:

· Heart disease
· Stroke
· Lung disease
· Diabetes

- Cancer
- Non-alcoholic fatty liver disease
- Gall bladder disease
- Osteoarthritis
- Pancreatitis

So how did this happen?

THE LINK BETWEEN DIET AND OBESITY

IN 1977 A U.S. Senate committee published a new set of dietary guidelines for Americans. Today, the U.S. Department of Health and Human Services and the U.S. Department of Agriculture (USDA) update and publish a new set every five years. To battle heart disease, which was the primary health concern in the 1970s, the guidelines recommended significant cuts to people's consumption of dietary fat. Even as people became obese, these same guidelines were trotted out to do battle with this new enemy. The original 1980 food pyramid from the USDA suggested that Americans eat 6 to 11 servings of refined grains, such as bread, cereal, rice, and pasta *every single day*. I'm not sure that I know anybody who considers eating 11 slices of white bread daily to be a slimming diet. Yet this was the very diet recommended by the government of the United States and followed by other countries around the world. Virtually every health professional, doctor, and dietician in the world was soon giving this advice.

In addition to low-fat diets, the other big trend of the 1970s was the increase in leisure-time exercise. Before then, the idea of exercising for health or fun was as foreign as rap music to disco fans. Originally this advice was given to improve heart health, leading to a boom in "cardio" exercises such as aerobics and running. This advice was soon co-opted for weight loss as well, despite the utter lack of evidence supporting the efficacy of these exercise programs for weight loss.

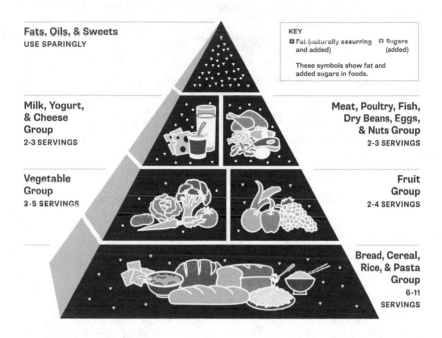

Figure 4.2. The U.S. Department of Agriculture's 1992 food pyramid[3]

Today, there are more gyms per capita than ever before. Local marathons and 10K races attract tens of thousands of runners. For most of her life, my grandmother never saw a gym. While exercise certainly has many health benefits (improved muscle tone, improved flexibility, increased bone mass, etc.), *weight loss is not one of them.* Scientific studies repeatedly confirm the minimal weight-loss effect of exercise programs. Two main reasons explain why. First, doing more exercise generally leads to eating more food, which will negate much of the weight-loss effects. They don't say that you are "working up an appetite" for no reason. Second, doing more exercise reduces a person's overall activity at other times of the day. For example, if you work a physically demanding job like construction for eight hours every day, then it is unlikely you will get home and decide to go on a 10K run just for fun. If you have been sitting in front of a computer all day, then that 10K run may sound quite appealing, but increasing leisure time exercise does not change total daily activity.

From the 1970s on, we have continued to believe that a low-fat diet combined with exercise will reduce weight and that people who are obese are just lacking in willpower. What we now know is that while what we eat does affect our weight, dietary fat is not the culprit. To understand why, we need to look at what happens to food when it enters the body.

DIGESTION: HOW THE BODY BREAKS DOWN FOOD

ALL FOODS ARE a combination of three major components called macronutrients:

1. Proteins
2. Dietary fats
3. Carbohydrates

In turn, each macronutrient is composed of smaller units or building blocks.

Proteins are chains of building blocks called amino acids. In the human body there are at least 20 amino acids, which can be combined to form thousands of different proteins. Nine amino acids are considered essential because the human body cannot synthesize them, which means they must be obtained through diet. If you don't eat enough of these proteins, you will become malnourished. Food sources of protein include meats, poultry, and seafood; dairy milk, cheese, and yogurt; eggs; beans and legumes.

Dietary fats are molecules called triglycerides, which are composed of a glycerol backbone and three fatty acids. Certain types of fat are also considered essential and must be obtained through diet. These include the omega-3 and omega-6 fatty acids. Food sources of fats include oily fish; dairy milk, cheese, and yogurt; eggs; nuts and seeds; coconuts; avocados.

Carbohydrates are chains of sugars such as glucose, fructose, or lactose. Table sugar, called sucrose, is composed of one molecule of glucose linked to one molecule of fructose. Starches, like flour, are composed of long chains of glucose in the form of amylopectin or amylose. There are no essential carbohydrates. Food sources of carbohydrates include grains; fruits and vegetables; beans and legumes; energy drinks and alcohol.

Food also contains microscopic amounts of vitamins (A, B, C, D, E, K, etc.) and minerals (iron, copper, selenium, etc.), which are known as micronutrients.

Digestion is the process of breaking down macronutrients—proteins, dietary fats, and carbohydrates—into their smaller components for absorption by the body. The amino acids and fatty acids that make up proteins and fats, respectively, can be either used as building blocks for cell components or burned for energy. The sugars that make up carbohydrates are burned for energy, but they are not used to build other cell parts.

The chemical reactions involved in creating this energy and building cell parts are collectively called metabolism. And each macronutrient is metabolized differently. Why is this important? Because these differences affect how energy is stored and used.

Protein metabolism

Protein, like lean meat, is broken down into its component amino acids during digestion and transported to the liver. Amino acids are mainly used to rebuild proteins in blood cells, bone, muscle, connective tissue, skin, etc. Think of this process as being similar to taking the letters from a Scrabble board and reshuffling them to create new words. We eat animal and plant proteins, break them into amino acids, and then recombine them to form our own proteins.

The primary function of ingested protein is to rebuild cell components, and burning it for energy is only a secondary function. If you eat more protein than is needed for rebuilding, there is no way to store these extra amino acids. Instead, the liver changes them into glucose by a process called gluconeogenesis, or "the formation of new glucose." (This word is derived from "gluco" meaning "glucose," "neo" meaning "new," and "genesis" meaning "the formation of.") For an average American adult, an estimated 50 to 70 percent of ingested protein is turned into glucose for energy.[4] However, this percentage varies greatly depending upon your body weight and how much protein you are eating.

Dietary protein takes significant processing by gluconeogenesis before it is converted to glucose. By this time, the body has activated multiple hormonal systems to deal with the expected increase in glucose availability. Thus, blood glucose remains stable even if you eat lots of protein.

Insulin is released when eating protein, especially in patients with type 2 diabetes, and signals the cell to start synthesizing new proteins. Certain animal proteins, such as the whey in dairy, generate almost as much of an insulin response as carbohydrates.

Fat metabolism

Digestion of dietary fat requires bile to mix and emulsify it. Bile is secreted by the liver, stored in the gallbladder, and released by the small intestine. Once the fat is absorbed by the small intestine, it is in droplets known as chylomicrons that are absorbed into the lymphatic system, which empties directly into the bloodstream. These chylomicrons are carried to fat cells called adipocytes, where they deliver a form of fat called triglycerides that are taken up for storage.

Dietary fat is absorbed more or less directly into our stores of body fat. While it may appear that dietary fat is far more conducive to increasing overall body fat, we will see later that this is not the case.

Carbohydrate metabolism

The chains of glucose found in carbohydrates are digested or broken into smaller units of glucose for absorption by the body. The speed of digestion and absorption depends upon many factors. Refined carbohydrates, such as grains like rice that have been husked or polished, are absorbed almost instantly because processing removes most of the associated fiber, proteins, and fats that slow absorption.

Unrefined carbohydrates, such as beans and legumes, are absorbed more slowly because none of the fiber or protein has been removed. Also, grinding grains like wheat into a very fine flour increases the speed of absorption.

The specific type of carbohydrate also makes a difference. Wheat contains mainly amylopectin A, which is quickly and easily absorbed by the body. In contrast, beans and legumes are high in amylopectin C, which resists digestion by the human body and is incompletely absorbed. The amylopectin C that remains in the intestines is eaten by the gut microbiome, which produces gas and is responsible for the flatulence associated with these pulses.

Blood glucose rises quickly when eating refined carbohydrates, stimulating secretion of the hormone insulin from the pancreas. The insulin sends a signal that moves glucose into cells to be burned for energy. With glucose stored in the body's cells, blood glucose levels return to normal.

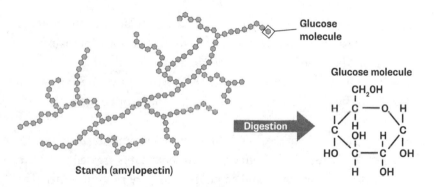

Figure 4.3. Carbohydrate metabolism

THE FED STATE: HOW THE BODY STORES FOOD ENERGY

THE BODY HAS two complementary methods of energy storage:

1. Glycogen (in the liver)
2. Body fat (in the fat cells)

When you eat more carbohydrates or proteins than your body needs, insulin rises. As we've seen, these macronutrients are converted into glucose and sent into the bloodstream, which causes your blood glucose levels to rise. This increase in blood glucose signals your pancreas to produce insulin, which indicates the availability of food and puts the body into the "fed" state. All the cells of the body (liver, kidney, brain, heart, muscles, etc.) can now help themselves to this all-you-can-eat glucose buffet.

If some glucose is left over, it must be stored away for future use. This is a relatively simple process, since the body just links all the glucose molecules into a long, branched chain called glycogen and stores it in the liver. Glycogen is made and stored directly in the liver. Our muscles also store their own supply of glycogen, but this source can only be used by the muscles. In other words, the glycogen within muscles cannot be used, for example, by the kidneys. In contrast, the glycogen in the liver can supply any organ by releasing glucose into the bloodstream.

In the fed state, insulin goes up, signaling the body to store excess food energy as glycogen. Liver-glycogen stores, if full, last approximately 24 hours. When the body's glycogen stores are full, the body must use a second form of energy storage for unused glucose. The excess glucose from the liver is converted into triglycerides, or body fat, through a process called "de novo lipogenesis," or creation of new fat. (The word "de novo" means "from new" and "lipogenesis" means "creation of new fat.") Some of the glucose from which this body fat is created may have come from carbohydrates and some from dietary protein, which was changed from protein to glucose through gluconeogenesis.

Regardless of where the excess glucose comes from, the liver creates new fat (triglycerides) but cannot store it. Fat is designed to be stored in fat cells (adipocytes), not the liver. So the liver packages these triglycerides together with some transport proteins and exports them as very low-density lipoprotein (VLDL). In the bloodstream, insulin increases a hormone known as lipoprotein lipase (LPL), which helps the triglycerides move out of the VLDL particle and into the adipocyte. This effectively transforms excess glucose into triglycerides and moves them to the appropriate fat cells for long-term storage. If the rate of new fat creation from de novo lipogenesis exceeds the export capacity of the liver, these triglycerides back up in the liver and cause non-alcoholic fatty liver disease.

Remember, this process is not the same as ingesting dietary fat. The fat we eat is broken down into chylomicrons, absorbed by the small intestine, and sent directly into the adipocytes. There is no processing within the liver, no insulin signaling, and no possibility of using the glycogen storage system, which is exclusively for glucose.

This entire storage process for fat is much more laborious compared with the relatively simple glycogen storage. So why have the two different systems? The glycogen and body fat systems for storing food energy complement each other perfectly. Glycogen is easy to get to and convenient, but limited in storage space. Body fat is harder to get to and inconvenient, but unlimited in storage space.

Think of glycogen like a wallet. You can move your cash into and out of your wallet without much difficulty, but you would not hold six months' worth of cash in your wallet. Think of body fat like your bank account. It is more difficult to move money back and forth: you have to go to a bank machine or teller, put money in, and perhaps buy investments. Getting your money out as cash is also not so simple, because you need to go back to the bank to withdraw it. But you can store your life's savings in a bank account without worry. This balance between short-term and long-term storage in the body also applies when you want to use that stored energy, as we'll see next.

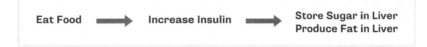

Figure 4.4. How the body stores food energy (calories)

THE FASTED STATE: HOW THE BODY
USES STORED FOOD ENERGY

THE WORD "FASTING" may sound scary, but it simply refers to any time you are not eating. When you sleep, for example, you are fasting. In the fasted state, your body reverses its process for storing food. When insulin falls, as with fasting, the body breaks glycogen back down into individual glucose molecules to supply energy to the whole body. This is why we don't die in our sleep every single night. "Breakfast" is literally the meal that breaks our fast, so you can see that fasting is a part of everyday life.

Put another way, at any given time our bodies exist in only one of two states: the fed state or the fasted state. Our body is either storing food energy or using it up. High insulin is the body's signal to store incoming food energy. Low insulin is the body's signal to use the stored food energy because no food is coming in. In the fasted state, we must rely on our stores of food energy to survive.

First, the body breaks glycogen down into glucose that can be burned for energy. This supply lasts approximately 24 hours if the glycogen stores are full. If you fast for more than 24 hours, the body turns to the harder-to-access stores of body fat. Thinking in terms of the bank analogy, once you use up the cash in your wallet, you will need to turn to your harder-to-access bank account or safety deposit box for more money. In other words, glycogen is the better solution for short-term energy needs, and body fat is the better solution for longer-term needs. This partially explains why it is so difficult to lose body fat. It is easier for somebody to steal cash from the wallet (glycogen) in your jacket pocket than to steal the investments or gold bars locked away in your bank's safety deposit box (body fat). Understanding how to access these energy stores is crucial to understanding how to lose weight.

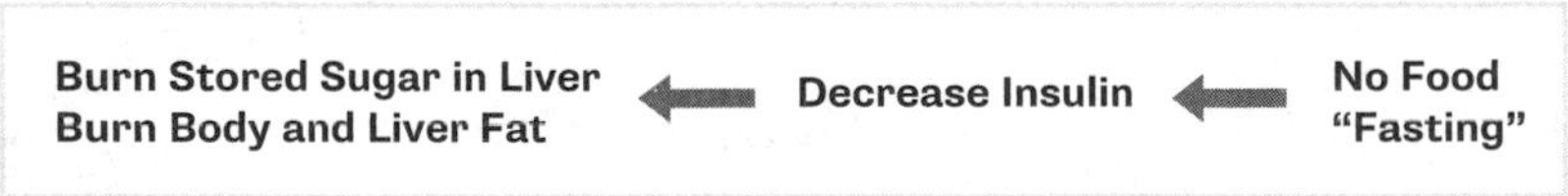

Burn Stored Sugar in Liver Burn Body and Liver Fat	⬅	Decrease Insulin	⬅	No Food "Fasting"

Figure 4.5. How the body burns food energy (calories)

If you eat a diet that is very low in carbohydrates, moderate in proteins, and high in natural fats, sometimes called a ketogenic diet, your glycogen stores will be low. Remember, only dietary carbohydrates and excess proteins can be stored as glycogen. If you have no glycogen to burn for energy, the body must burn its fat reserves to fulfill its energy needs.

A healthy body exists in the balance between feeding and fasting. There are times that you should store food energy and times that you should burn it. Too much of one or the other will result in illness. Balancing the fed and fasted states keeps body weight stable.

Insulin levels are the crucial factor in determining whether we store food energy or burn it. In technical terms, we say that insulin inhibits lipolysis (the breakdown of fat), a fact we've known for at least 50 years. In lay terms, we can say that insulin blocks fat burning. High insulin levels keep your body in the fed state, which means storing food energy rather than burning it. In contrast, low insulin allows access to body fat.

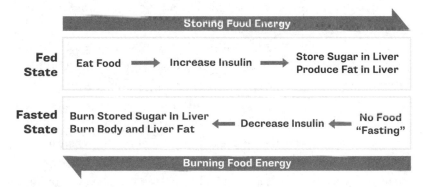

Figure 4.6. The fed state versus the fasted state

HORMONES: A NEW WAY TO THINK ABOUT WEIGHT GAIN AND WEIGHT LOSS

AFTER 50 YEARS of desperate, intense research, guess how many studies prove the effectiveness of counting calories for weight loss? Zero. That's right: *Nada. Zilch.* Zero. The scientific evidence proves the complete failure of this strategy of caloric reduction as primary goal. That's because the key to successful weight loss is to control your body's "thermostat," the body set weight (BSW).

In your home, the thermostat keeps your room at a perfect temperature despite wildly varying outside conditions. When the temperature is hot outside, the thermostat turns on the air conditioning. When the thermostat detects the temperature is too cold, it turns on the heat. In our bodies, we have the BSW, also called an appestat or obesistat, which is essentially a thermostat for body fatness.

Satiety hormones

Some people believe we are designed to eat everything in front of our faces, and now that food is so easily available, we have no choice but to gain weight. This is completely false. The truth is that we have powerful, overlapping satiety mechanisms to stop eating. We have stretch receptors in our stomach to signal when it is too full. We have powerful satiety hormones such as peptide YY and cholecystokinin that stop us from eating.

From an evolutionary standpoint, these satiety mechanisms make a lot of sense. Our body is designed to stay within certain body fat parameters. If you are too skinny, you will die during times when food is scarce. If you are too fat, you will not be able to catch food and you might just get eaten yourself. Wild animals almost never become obese to the point of being unable to function normally. Where are the morbidly obese antelope? Caribou? Lions? Tigers? Fish? When food is plentiful, the numbers of animals increase, not the size of individual animals. For example, you don't get a few morbidly obese rats. You get thousands of relatively normal-sized rats.

Insulin: The energy storage and energy use hormone

The BSW sets an ideal body fatness that it defends just like our house thermostat. If you are too skinny, your body tries to gain weight. If you are too fat, your body tries to lose weight. The clearest experimental demonstration of this effect was done by Dr. Rudy Leibel in 1995. In this experiment, he took volunteers and overfed them to make them gain 10 percent more weight. Then he returned them to their regular weight, and then to 10 or 20 percent weight loss. At each point, he measured the basal metabolic rate (BMR), or how much energy (calories) the body is expending.

After 10 percent weight gain, the participants' bodies burned about 500 calories more per day compared with baseline. The body was trying to burn off the excess calories to return to its BSW. When participants returned to their original weight, so did their metabolic rate. After 10 percent weight loss, they burned about 300 fewer calories per day. Once again, the body was trying very hard to maintain its BSW in the original position, acting just like our house thermostat.

The body seeks homeostasis, which is why counting calories is futile. The body can burn more or fewer calories depending upon the situation. The hormone insulin instructs the body to gain body fat. If you are not eating enough, you will become hungry so that the body can obey its directive. If that still does not work, then the body will reduce its use of energy so the available calories can be stored as body fat. When that happens, your BMR slows, your body burns fewer calories, and your weight loss will stall.

Insulin is the main controller of the body fatness thermostat. If you keep feeding the body, it will continue to gain body fat. Insulin will keep directing the body to convert the food energy to glycogen and body fat. This is the reason that continual snacking leads to weight gain. It is also the reason that insulin injections lead to weight gain. Your body has no mechanism to count calories. In fact, it doesn't give a hoot about them. And if your body doesn't count calories, why should you?

WATCH YOUR HORMONES, NOT YOUR CALORIES

NEED MORE CONVINCING? Consider two foods of equal caloric value. On the one hand you have 200 calories of cookies, and on the other, 200 calories of salmon. The number of calories is identical. When you eat either of those two foods, does your body somehow measure the calories? No, your body has no idea how many calories are in each food. Are these two foods of identical calories equally fattening? No! Nobody believes that eating cookies is equal to eating salmon.

So why does eating cookies cause more weight gain than eating salmon? Remember what we said about how carbohydrates, proteins, and dietary fats are digested by the body. Is the metabolic effect on the body the same for each of these equal-calorie foods? *Absolutely not.* As soon as we start digesting, the body's response is completely and utterly different.

Cookies, which are refined carbohydrates, will strongly stimulate insulin. They will not activate any of the powerful satiety hormones such as peptide YY and cholecystokinin that stop us from eating. Eating cookies will not satisfy your hunger. Salmon, on the other hand, has entirely different metabolic effects. Insulin goes up, but much, much less than with the cookies. The protein and fat will activate satiety hormones and make you feel full. That is why—after eating too much at an all-you-can-eat buffet—you can still eat a few cookies for dessert. Could you eat another small piece of salmon? The mere thought may make you nauseous.

What the body cares about are the hormones signaling us to eat or not eat, and the hormones telling us to store fat or burn fat. This is the very reason that artificial, noncaloric sweeteners have entirely failed to halt the obesity epidemic. If the most important determinant of body fatness was the number of calories we consume, we could simply eat fake sugar, fake fat, and other fake foods that contain no calories. Then we would lose weight and live happily ever after. But that hasn't happened.

All foods raise insulin to some degree, so there will be an overlap between the number of calories and the insulin effect. Foods that strongly stimulate insulin are more fattening (cookies) than those that do not (salmon). But this simply means that some foods are more fattening than others. It doesn't mean that calories are a useful concept in weight loss.

To understand weight loss, we need to understand what our body cares about. The answer is hormones, mostly insulin. So what does this tell us about PCOS?

Insulin: The Common Link between PCOS and Obesity

....

LIKE PCOS, AN estimated 70 percent of obesity may be related to genetics. Both tend to run in families. However, not all obese women have PCOS, and not all women with PCOS are obese. I am a great example. Nevertheless, obesity is one of the most common—and perhaps most important—features of PCOS, despite the fact that it is not part of the diagnostic criteria. Obesity occurs in 30 to 75 percent of women with PCOS[1] and is associated with the worsening of all three primary diagnostic features of PCOS—increased masculinizing features, worsening menstrual difficulties, and more ovarian cysts. In women with PCOS, the risk of prediabetes and type 2 diabetes increases as body weight increases.

There is an obvious connection, but the exact link is under debate. There are three possibilities to consider:

· PCOS causes obesity.
· Obesity causes PCOS.
· Both obesity and PCOS are caused by a third problem.

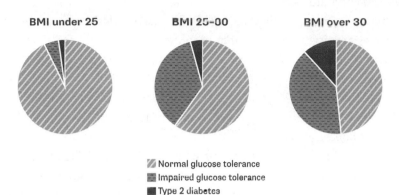

BMI under 25   **BMI 25-00**   **BMI over 30**

%// Normal glucose tolerance
☰ Impaired glucose tolerance
■ Type 2 diabetes

Figure 5.1. Prevalence (%) by Body Mass Index (kg/m²) of glucose intolerance in American women with PCOS[?]

DOES PCOS CAUSE OBESITY?

WHILE PREPUBERTAL GIRLS and boys have roughly the same percentage of body fat, this changes dramatically during puberty. Increased testosterone in young men causes less fat accumulation than the increased estrogens in females. Under the influence of estrogens, girls will gain approximately 50 percent more body fat than boys. The fat is also distributed to the hips and breasts in females, as opposed to the more central distribution in males. The difference in the distribution of fat between males and females that appears shortly after puberty also disappears after menopause.

During the period in which women have more body fat than men, the distribution of that fat is important. Women without PCOS have more subcutaneous (under the skin) fat on their arms and legs than concentrated in the abdominal area. High testosterone, which is associated with hyperandrogenism, promotes central, or visceral, obesity, where the fat is distributed primarily in and around the abdominal organs.

An estimated 50 to 60 percent of women with PCOS have central obesity, *regardless of their BMI*. This fat distribution is often noticeable as an increased waist circumference and it is also referred to as "masculinized body fat distribution,"[3] which is associated with lower conception rates and ovulatory frequency. The heavier a woman gets, the less likely she is to ovulate. Central obesity is also a far greater risk factor for metabolic syndrome and cardiovascular disease than other types of obesity.

Although obesity is associated with PCOS, none of the diagnostic conditions—polycystic ovaries, anovulation, and hyperandrogenism— causes obesity. The excess androgens affect only the distribution of fat, not the increase in overall body fat.

DOES OBESITY CAUSE PCOS?

THAT IS A more interesting possibility. The severity and risk of developing PCOS increase with obesity but the correlation is very loose. In obesity clinics, a new diagnosis of PCOS was made in 28.3 percent of patients. This is a whopping five-fold increase over the 5.5 percent prevalence in lean women in the general population.[4]

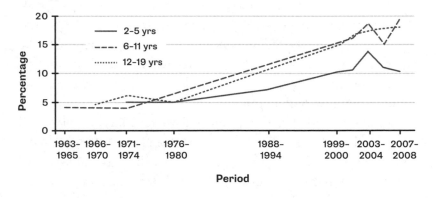

Figure 5.2. Prevalence of obesity among children and adolescents, by age group—United States, 1963–2008. Reproduced with permission of the Centers for Disease Control and Prevention. Use of this figure does not constitute endorsement by the CDC.[5]

In the United States, rates of childhood and adolescent obesity have almost quadrupled in the last 40 years. And obesity in childhood and adolescence is a well-known risk factor for PCOS. Obese adolescents with PCOS have higher insulin levels and increased insulin resistance, which emphasizes the huge role insulin plays in obesity.[6] In one study, 65 percent of obese prepubertal girls were found to have elevated testosterone levels, which shows the relationship between obesity and hyperandrogenism.[7]

Today, people are eating more processed foods, in greater amounts, more times per day. Fifty years ago, my grandmother ate two to three meals per day, all of them based on whole, unprocessed, mostly home-grown foods. Snacks? Forget about them. Today, my kids' pediatrician recommends I feed them six to seven small meals per day focusing on "whole grains, low-fat foods, and lots of fruit and vegetables." But these foods, respectively, are processed, processed, and partially modified. My kids' school has a "healthy snack program," yet it is bizarre to consider that snacking was considered a superfluous luxury only a generation ago and now it is considered a necessity. The truth is that humans have survived for thousands of years without snacking, and there is simply no medical requirement to put muffins in our mouths every few hours to be healthy. Though I still get notes from school "reminding" me that snacks are important and that it's a "long time" between breakfast and lunch, I resist the peer pressure because I know better.

Weight loss improves all signs and symptoms of PCOS. In one study, after bariatric (weight-loss) surgery, not only did patients lose weight but their hirsutism and androgen levels decreased, their insulin resistance resolved, and their irregular menstrual cycles became regular. The diagnosis of PCOS could not be sustained in any of the patients after surgery, showing that PCOS may potentially be reversed with weight loss.[8]

But obesity is clearly not the sole cause of PCOS, which I know from my own experience. Indeed, I was normal weight or even mildly underweight according to BMI at the time of my diagnosis, but I had clear evidence of PCOS. And though rates of obesity vary widely throughout the world, rates of PCOS do not. For example, the prevalence of PCOS is fairly similar in the United States, Spain, and the U.K., but obesity differs significantly among those countries. Studies show only a very loose correlation between the severity of the obesity and the prevalence of PCOS.[9] While increasingly severe obesity, as measured by BMI, is associated with higher rates of PCOS, the correlation is not tight enough to suggest a direct causal relationship.

In my own case, I gained 20 to 30 pounds (9 to 13.6 kilograms) in three months, which made me stop ovulating. The weight was wholly concentrated on my belly and nowhere else, and my BMI did not classify me as obese or even overweight. When I lost some of that weight on a very low-carb diet, I conceived the following month, yet before that I hadn't been able to spontaneously conceive after a year of trying. Obesity, while clearly related in some way to PCOS, is not the sole cause. This leaves only the third possibility, that some underlying factor causes both obesity and PCOS.

IS INSULIN THE COMMON LINK?

GIVEN THAT OBESITY is a hormonal imbalance that results in the gradual increase of the body set weight (BSW) thermostat over time, it is likely that the root cause of PCOS is also hormonal.

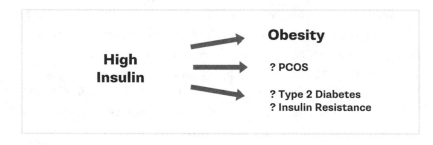

Figure 5.3. Is high insulin the root cause of metabolic disease?

But is insulin the other factor? In the study of a disease, the most crucial piece of information is its etiology, a medical term for what causes it. If you know that a virus causes hepatitis C, you can prescribe an antiviral that kills the virus and cures the disease. If you understand that smoking causes lung cancer, you can prevent much of this disease by introducing smoking-cessation programs. We can get a hint of PCOS's etiology by looking at its associated conditions. Let's start with hyperandrogenism.

6

Insulin and
Hyperandrogenism

....

A 24-YEAR-OLD WOMAN PRESENTED to her physicians with some unusual symptoms.[1] During exercise, she experienced a full grand mal seizure without any previous history of epilepsy. In the prior six months, she had become very tired and noted episodes of trembling, blurred vision, and confusion. She could control these symptoms by eating. Upon investigation, she was found to have a rare insulin-secreting tumor of the pancreas known as an insulinoma. This tumor was massively overproducing insulin, causing her blood sugar to fall very low after an overnight fast. She had way too much insulin in her system.

Upon further questioning, she also noted acne, hirsutism, and very irregular periods that had varied from 40 to 44 days over the previous year. An ultrasound revealed polycystic ovaries, and bloodwork revealed high testosterone levels. She was diagnosed with PCOS. She had a normal Body Mass Index and was not overweight. A scan revealed a three-quarter-inch (2-centimeter) tumor mass in her pancreas, and she underwent surgery to remove it. Four months after the operation, her menstrual cycles became regular at 28 days, she lost 8.8 pounds

(4 kilograms) of weight, and her acne and hirsutism fully resolved. Bloodwork revealed that her insulin level had normalized and along with it her testosterone levels. This case provides dramatic insight into the causal role of excessive insulin and PCOS as well as weight gain, which earlier studies had already hinted at.

EARLY RESEARCH INTO HYPERANDROGENISM AND HORMONES

THE HORMONAL UNDERPINNINGS of PCOS began to be appreciated in the 1950s, when the development of the radioimmunoassay made it possible to measure very small amounts of substances, including hormone levels, in the blood. In the 1960s and 1970s, research focused on luteinizing hormone (LH) and follicle-stimulating hormone (FSH), which are key regulators of the normal menstrual cycle. For many years, an abnormal LH/FSH ratio was considered diagnostic of PCOS. By the 1980s, testosterone was recognized as the main androgen responsible for the majority of PCOS-related problems[2]

Testosterone is produced normally in both the ovaries and the adrenal gland, a small gland that sits on top of the kidneys. In addition to androgens, the adrenal gland also produces other hormones, including cortisol, adrenalin, and aldosterone. So the next step was to figure out which organ—the ovaries or the adrenal glands—was responsible for the overproduction of testosterone in women with PCOS.

Normally, the ovaries and adrenal glands contribute equally to testosterone production. By 1989 studies showed that in women with PCOS, the ovary is the key source of excessive testosterone production. Specifically, it is the theca cells within the ovary that are responsible for the overproduction. In addition, Stein and Leventhal had revealed that surgically removing a wedge of the ovary (ovarian wedge resection) often restored normal ovulation and normal menstrual cycles. If the adrenal gland were responsible for overproducing androgens, cutting a little wedge out of the ovary would not make any difference. Therefore, it was concluded that the hyperandrogenism of PCOS was caused by an overproduction of testosterone secreted mostly by the ovaries. This hyperandrogenism, in turn, caused the symptoms of hirsutism and infertility.

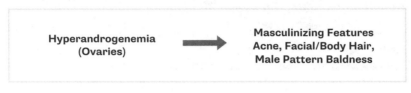

Figure 6.1. Excess androgens lead to masculinizing features

Hormones and the role of carrier proteins

Blood testosterone levels are not directly measured as part of the diagnostic criteria for PCOS because doing so is highly problematic. First, testosterone levels vary widely throughout the day and with age and menstrual status. Second, even in women with diagnosed PCOS, the ovarian portion of testosterone production only rises to about 60 percent of the total daily production of testosterone.[3] Third, a major contributing factor to the excess androgen effect seen in PCOS (hirsutism, acne, etc.) is not excessive testosterone but low levels of sex hormone–binding globulin (SHBG).

Hormones travel around the bloodstream bound up with other proteins that accompany them to their proper destination. Think of a hormone as a visitor to New York City for a business meeting. Even if you know the route, getting to your destination on foot is slow and it might be tempting to shop at stores along the way. Instead, a better solution is to find a taxi and travel directly to the meeting.

The SHBG protein is designed to accompany testosterone. Without its carrier protein SHBG, the unchaperoned testosterone, like other "free" hormones, would stop off at every tissue to exert its effects and never get to its intended destination. The testosterone produced in the ovary might stop by the liver, kidneys, and fat tissue before getting to the skin. So the SHBG ensures that it gets to its intended destination.

Most hormones in the human body have their own specific carrier protein. And many of these carrier proteins are called globulins because they are globular in shape. Thyroid hormone, for example, is only carried by thyroid-binding globulin (TBG). It cannot bind to, say, SHBG, which carries testosterone. So what happens if the proper carriers are not available?

Remember that unchaperoned testosterone? That hormone is like the visitor to New York City looking for a taxi just as a baseball game in Yankee Stadium finishes. There aren't enough taxis, and the 50,000 fans are just milling around the street going into all the stores and bars. It's overcrowded around Yankee Stadium, but their intended destinations (home) are all empty. Just like the fans wandering the streets around Yankee Stadium, testosterone floats around freely in the blood if there are not enough SHBG carrier proteins.

Testosterone in high levels starts to exert its masculinizing effects on the neighboring organs because it is not getting to its proper destination. Thus, you develop acne, excessive facial hair, and male-pattern baldness. The total amount of testosterone might be the same, but the lack of carrier protein, SHBG, allows the excessive effect of this androgen. In other words, the masculinizing features present in women with PCOS result not only because of too many androgens in the blood but because a lack of SHBG means they cannot get to their intended destination. What, then, causes the lack of SHBG? The answer is insulin.

THE INSULIN CONNECTION

INSULIN IS THE major regulator of SHBG production in the liver. The higher the insulin, the lower the SHBG production. This relationship holds true not just in women but also in men.[4] Decreasing insulin levels through weight loss increases SHBG production.

A population-based study in Sweden confirmed the inverse relationship.[5] Type 1 diabetics, who have very low insulin levels, had very high SHBG. Type 2 diabetics, who have very high insulin levels, had very low SHBG. Insulin directly reduces liver production of SHBG and therefore increases the levels of free and bioavailable androgens.

Thus, excessive insulin causes both

1. overproduction of testosterone and
2. decreased SHBG levels that lead to increased testosterone effect.

The striking correlation between blood levels of insulin and testosterone was noted as far back as 1980.[6] They showed an astounding 85 percent correlation with each other, and the fact that these two hormones were moving in almost exact lockstep is highly suggestive that one hormone was directly stimulating the other. The question was, Did high testosterone cause high insulin, or did high insulin cause high testosterone?

Elegant studies with isolated cell cultures clarified the connection.[7] When you purify ovarian cells and bathe them in insulin, they increase testosterone production significantly. The opposite is not true. If you bathe ovarian cells in testosterone, nothing happens, since the ovary does not produce insulin. The pancreas is responsible for insulin production and secretion. If you give testosterone to experimental subjects, insulin secretion by the pancreas does not change at all. Clearly, insulin drives testosterone production and not the other way around.

Human studies have confirmed that high insulin does indeed increase androgen levels. Direct insulin infusion measurably increases the levels of androgens.[8] Put more simply, the more insulin you give, the higher the testosterone production in the ovary. Even 24 hours after insulin infusion was stopped, the testosterone levels continued to be elevated.

The surprising link between insulin and reproduction

The ovary itself is particularly rich in insulin receptors,[9] which seems rather strange at first glance because insulin is most commonly associated with digestion, blood glucose, and body fat. Why would the ovaries carry insulin receptors? In fact, the pathways that link reproductive function and metabolism are seen in virtually every living animal, from fruit flies to roundworms to human beings. Why?

The answer is that all animals need to know that food is available before committing to reproduction. Raising children requires a good deal of resources, including adequate food supplies for both the expectant mother and the developing baby.

We know that adults can live on relatively low levels of food energy and nutrients. During World War II, when food was rationed or unavailable, for example, many people survived on what would now be considered woefully inadequate amounts of food. Adults require fewer nutrients because human organs do not grow once they reach adult size. In tough times, we can break down old liver cells to build new liver cells.

A baby, however, must eat enough nutrients to build new cells so its organs can develop and grow. A baby may enter the world weighing only 7 pounds (3 kilograms) but eventually grows to perhaps 150 pounds (68 kilograms). In addition to storing energy for normal cellular function, that baby must also gain 143 pounds (65 kilograms) of matter to build proteins, fat cells, internal organs, muscles, etc. This is a very resource-intensive labor of love.

If humans produce too many babies when food is scarce, neither the baby nor the mother will survive. Therefore, the ovary has evolved a mechanism to obtain reliable information about the availability of food in the outside world. It should only produce eggs when food is available to sustain the growth of the baby. But trapped inside the pelvis, without eyes, ears, or nose, how can the ovary gauge what's happening in the outside world? It uses nutrient sensors.

Insulin is one of those nutrient sensors. When you eat food, insulin rises, which signals that food is available. If the ovary's insulin receptors sense the presence of this hormone, it proceeds with normal egg development. But if too much insulin is available, then the process goes awry.

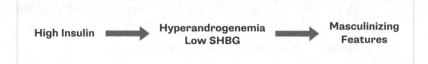

Figure 6.2. High insulin is the root cause of masculinizing features

We've seen that high insulin increases testosterone and decreases SHBG, thereby causing the masculinizing features associated with PCOS. To confirm that conclusion, several studies have shown that using diazoxide to block insulin[10] or drugs such as metformin or thiazolidinediones to lower insulin effectively decreases testosterone levels. In contrast, surgically removing part of the ovaries in women with PCOS reverses the hyperandrogenism but not the high insulin levels.[11]

We can conclude, therefore, that a high insulin level is the primary factor stimulating excessive ovarian production of testosterone and that this increased androgen (hyperandrogenism) is responsible for the masculinizing features of PCOS, including acne and hirsutism.[12] Hyperinsulinemia, too much insulin in the blood, is the root cause of hyperandrogenism. Too much insulin causes too much testosterone. Is insulin responsible for the lack of ovulation and polycystic ovaries too?

Insulin, Polycystic Ovaries, and Anovulation

....

MICHELLE WAS ONE of my first patients when I returned to practice in Toronto in 2014. At the time, she was a morbidly obese young lady in her early twenties. She had been diagnosed with PCOS in her early teens and hadn't had a menstrual cycle for three years. The physical signs of PCOS were obvious: she had coarse, stubbly hair on her face and very thin hair on her scalp. Michelle's main concern when she came to see me was her weight.

I started Michelle on a very low-carbohydrate diet. Michelle never truly understood the science behind the low-carb diet, but she was very determined to lose weight so she went "all in." She loved the fact that following the diet was easy: she loved the food choices, she felt full at the end of a meal, and she didn't have to count calories. Most of all, she loved the fact that she was losing weight for the first time *ever*. She had been on and off diets her whole life, and her newfound success was hugely motivating.

Only three months later, Michelle had a menstrual cycle. She was not happy about it because she suffered the premenstrual symptoms of bloating and irritability, and her period "came with a vengeance," she said. She was acting like a teenager, I thought. If Michelle were a bit older and trying desperately to conceive, how would she have felt about *finally* getting a period after so many years of not ovulating? But Michelle's weight loss and her low-carb diet had seemingly restored her regular reproductive functioning, despite the PCOS diagnosis. To understand why, let's look at how the ovaries work and what causes the cysts for which this syndrome is named.

NORMAL FOLLICULAR DEVELOPMENT

FEMALES ARE BORN with ovaries that contain a finite pool of cells called primordial follicles, which have the potential to develop into a mature egg. From birth to menarche, all these primordial follicles remain dormant. At puberty, however, each month some of these primordial follicles are recruited for growth into primary follicles during the menstrual cycle. As women age, the number of follicles gradually decreases, as used follicles are never replaced. When the follicles are fully depleted, women undergo menopause and can no longer have children.

At the start of each menstrual cycle, a few primordial follicles grow into primary and then secondary follicles. Only one of these follicles is selected to become the dominant follicle. The rest simply involute (shrivel away) and are reabsorbed by the body. The dominant follicle alone continues to grow. At ovulation, in response to a surge in luteinizing hormone (LH), the egg is expelled into the respective fallopian tube, which carries it to the uterus. The rest of the dominant follicle becomes the corpus luteum, which secretes estrogen and progesterone to support the hoped-for pregnancy.

The key signal for a primary follicle to grow is testosterone. Insulin is important too, but it acts indirectly by increasing testosterone (see chapter 6).[1] Primary follicles are generally detectable by ultrasound when they reach 2 millimeters in size, and the dominant follicle typically measures 22 to 24 millimeters.

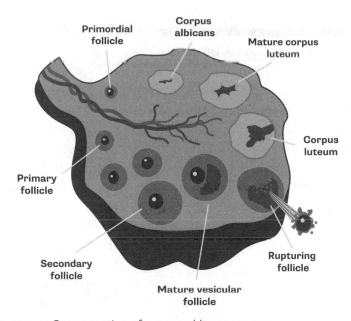

Figure 7.1. Cross-section of a normal human ovary

While the follicle is growing, the lining of the uterus thickens in preparation for the egg since it must supply all the necessary nutrients to await arrival of the sperm. If the sperm makes contact and fertilization occurs (yeah, baby), then the uterus continues to grow to sustain the developing fetus. This is the missed period that often signals a normal pregnancy. If the sperm (working late at the office) never arrives, then the egg cannot wait forever. The lining of the uterus is shed, along with the discarded egg, and a woman's period begins. Typically, this happens once a month.

The normal maturation process from primordial to primary to dominant follicle and then ovulation is quite orderly. Just as children start in kindergarten, work their way through one academic grade after another, and eventually graduate from high school, follicles start young and grow in an orderly fashion until finally, when mature, the egg is pushed out into the fallopian tube (ovulation) to await the sperm for fertilization.

FOLLICULAR ARREST: WHEN THE
MATURATION PROCESS GOES AWRY

IN 1982 IT was first observed that the ovaries of women with PCOS contain two to three times the number of primary follicles measuring 2 to 5 mm.[2] More recent studies suggest up to six times the usual number. The small ovarian follicles are rich in testosterone receptors, and it was determined that high testosterone levels were forcing too many primordial follicles from the resting phase to become primary follicles.[3]

Excessive testosterone has the same effect in other species and in women without PCOS who have high levels of testosterone. For example, experiments in rhesus monkeys show that administering high testosterone doses increases the number of primary follicles by three to five times. Testosterone therapy given to human female-to-male transgender people has the same effect. And women with rare testosterone-secreting adrenal tumors show the same abnormally high number of small follicles. There is a tight relationship between blood levels of testosterone and the number of follicles detected by ultrasound.

The problems don't stop there for people with PCOS. There are too many primary follicles but no single dominant follicle is selected to continue growing, which is the normal signal for the others to involute. The many small follicles don't shrivel up when they're supposed to, eventually fill with fluid (becoming cysts), and become visible as polycystic ovaries. This failure of the follicles to mature is called follicular arrest.

In women with PCOS, too many follicles start the transition from quiescent primordial follicle to growing primary follicle. But these follicles never grow up, and they never shrivel up either. In our school-child analogy, it is like starting six times the usual number of students in kindergarten and then having all of them stop their studies at sixth grade, never moving past that stage.

In PCOS, the many small follicles do not mature to become eggs that can be pushed out into the uterus for fertilization. This failure of ovulation causes the anovulatory cycles and menstrual irregularities.

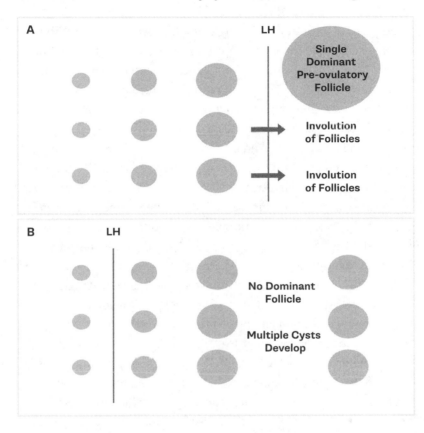

Figure 7.2. (A) Normal development of dominant follicle versus (B) follicular arrest caused by hyperinsulinemia initiating a premature response to luteinizing hormone (LH)[4]

THE INSULIN CONNECTION

. . . .

HIGH INSULIN LEVELS are predominantly responsible for the follicular arrest[5] by disturbing the delicately balanced ratio of follicle-stimulating hormone (FSH) to LH that triggers the correct follicular development.[6] During normal development, FSH encourages the growth of primordial follicles into primary follicles, and a surge of LH selects the dominant follicle, which leads to proper ovulation.

In women with PCOS, the high insulin levels promote the transition of primordial follicles to primary follicles.[7] They also increase testosterone levels, making the receptors on the primary follicles overly sensitive to LH. The primary follicles respond too early in the menstrual cycle and stop growing when they are still small and not yet ready for ovulation. Consequently, no single dominant follicle is selected and no signal is given for involution. The many small follicles simply accumulate fluid, and it is these numerous small fluid-filled cysts that are visible on ultrasound and clinch the diagnosis of PCOS.

In the school analogy, insulin is like a graduation letter sent to students so they can join the workforce or go to university. Under normal circumstances, this letter goes to twelfth-grade graduates who have had a full education and are old enough to leave school and live on their own. If these graduation letters are sent after sixth grade, the students will stop their schooling but they aren't ready to leave with a high school education and nor do they drop out of school. They just mill about the school building.

In women with PCOS, insulin sends its "stop growing" message to the follicles much too early. These immature follicles cannot be expelled as mature eggs and nor can they shrivel up. Eventually they become cysts. Lots and lots of cysts. Insulin causes this follicular arrest, which results in polycystic ovaries.

The eponymous criterion of PCOS is the presence of multiple cysts in the ovaries, which are derived from the multitude of small follicles. Many women have a few cysts in their ovaries, but the sheer number of cysts distinguishes this syndrome from virtually all others. Almost no other human disease causes polycystic ovaries. Ultimately, these polycystic ovaries are caused by too much insulin and too much testosterone.

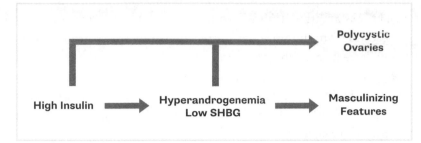

Figure 7.3. High insulin levels lead to both polycystic ovaries and masculinizing features

Both the cysts in the ovaries and the hyperandrogenism are caused by the same underlying problem—too much insulin. What about the other major criteria—the irregular menstrual cycles?

THE RELATIONSHIP BETWEEN POLYCYSTIC OVARIES, ANOVULATION, AND INSULIN

DURING FOLLICULAR ARREST, no dominant follicle grows large enough to ovulate. The result is a menstrual cycle in which no ovulation occurs (anovulatory cycle). No ovulation, no egg, no baby.

During the normal menstrual cycle, estrogen builds up the lining of the uterus. After ovulation, the remnant of the dominant follicle produces the hormone progesterone to prepare the uterus for pregnancy. Without ovulation, progesterone levels are low. The estrogen keeps building up the lining of the uterus, but a lack of progesterone prevents it from shedding (missed periods) until it eventually releases under its own weight (heavy bleeding). This leads to the irregular menstrual cycles associated with PCOS.

Almost all women will experience a few anovulatory cycles in their lifetimes, especially during puberty and menopause. However, the excessive insulin and testosterone in PCOS cause recurrent anovulatory cycles. Since testosterone is overproduced due to high insulin, the single most important cause of anovulatory cycles is high insulin. Both weight loss and the insulin-lowering drug metformin lower plasma testosterone and improve ovulatory rates.[8] Indeed, all known treatments to reduce insulin, including weight loss, bariatric surgery, and the drugs somatostatin and metformin, significantly improve ovulatory function and reduce the symptoms of PCOS. Interestingly, patients with type 1 diabetes who use high doses of injected insulin also have an increased risk of PCOS.

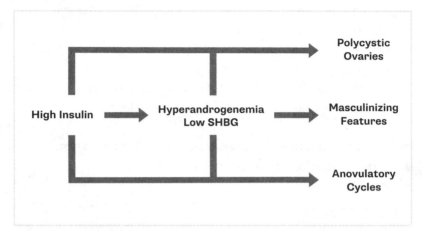

Figure 7.4. High insulin levels lead to all the features of PCOS

The bottom line, then, is that three defining features of PCOS—hyperandrogenism causing masculine features, polycystic ovaries, and anovulatory cycles—all reflect the same pathophysiology: too much testosterone, ultimately caused by too much insulin.

Simply put, too much insulin causes PCOS. Like obesity, PCOS is best understood as a disease of hyperinsulinemia. Although obesity and PCOS do not always occur together, they are both manifestations of an underlying hyperinsulinemia. So what is causing the high insulin levels?

8

Understanding the Roots of Insulin Resistance

....

I N 1976 A landmark paper was published in the prestigious *New England Journal of Medicine* describing a 13-year-old girl with extreme insulin resistance. She suffered from a rare genetic condition now known to be Donohue Syndrome, or leprechaunism, a genetic defect of the insulin receptor.[1]

Hormones are chemical messengers that interact with cells much like a lock and key. Under normal conditions, the hormone insulin (the key) must fit into a cell's proper receptor (the lock) in order to open a gate that allows glucose into the cell. If either the key or the lock is defective, the gate will not open. In leprechaunism, the insulin receptor is defective so the only solution is to give lots of insulin to force the lock and allow glucose into cells. The girl described in the paper required a massive 48,000 units of insulin per day to survive. By comparison, healthy humans produce 15 to 20 units of insulin per day, and even severe type 2 diabetics usually take less than 100 units per day.

These large doses of insulin caused hirsutism, acanthosis nigricans (a dark, velvety rash of the skin commonly associated with high insulin levels), and bilaterally enlarged ovaries—all features of PCOS. In effect, huge insulin doses were creating too much testosterone, which caused PCOS.

A study that followed patients with high insulin levels for 30 years showed that hyperandrogenism is a clear consequence of these high insulin levels.[2] Insulin relentlessly drives androgen production in the ovaries, to the point that many patients required surgical removal of their ovaries or wedge resections to remove some of the ovaries in order to control their symptoms. This was the same procedure used in 1935 by Drs. Stein and Leventhal.

As a result of these findings, researchers wondered if all women with PCOS show evidence of hyperinsulinemia and insulin resistance. Their hunch turned out to be correct.

HYPERINSULINEMIA, INSULIN RESISTANCE, AND PCOS

ALL KNOWN FORMS of insulin resistance are associated with PCOS. By 1980 hyperinsulinemia and insulin resistance were noted in obese PCOS patients,[3] were unusually severe in patients with PCOS compared with a non-PCOS population, and were out of proportion to the degree of obesity.[4]

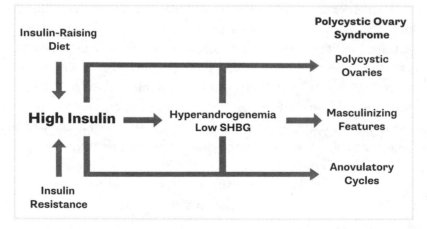

Figure 8.1. Both an insulin-raising diet and insulin resistance contribute to high insulin levels

The conclusion is that high blood insulin levels (hyperinsulinemia) drive PCOS. Moreover, the phenomenon known as insulin resistance *causes* hyperinsulinemia. Insulin resistance is a factor in type 2 diabetes and a risk factor for metabolic syndrome. It is this association with hyperinsulinemia and insulin resistance that firmly established PCOS as a metabolic disorder and accounts for the increased prevalence of type 2 diabetes, central adiposity, and metabolic disease in women with PCOS. Metabolic syndrome affects an estimated one-third of adolescents and half of all adults with PCOS.[5]

Hyperinsulinemia means too much insulin in the blood. Insulin resistance means that even though insulin levels are normal or high, glucose remains in the blood outside cells. Insulin should signal cells to allow glucose entry, but they "resist" the order. The cells in two organs—the muscles and liver—take up 85 percent of the glucose when stimulated by insulin[6] and thus account for most of the insulin resistance.

But there's a paradox here. Hyperinsulinemia stimulates the secretion of testosterone in the ovaries and lowers the production of sex hormone–binding globulin (SHBG) in the liver, which thus causes PCOS. But if the body is resistant to all of insulin's effect, then why are the ovary and the liver still responding correctly to insulin's signal to produce more testosterone and less SHBG? When people refer to insulin resistance, they are only referring to the effect on glucose's entry into cells, and not to any of the other effects of insulin. Why would insulin do one part of its job correctly but not the other?

Selective insulin resistance and the fallacy of internal cell starvation

In women with PCOS, both insulin and its receptor are demonstrably normal. That is, both the key and the lock are undamaged. For a long time, researchers imagined that glucose was not making it into the cell because the gate was closed and something was gumming up the mechanism to make it malfunction. They believed that glucose levels inside the cell were low. Although they could not directly measure these internal glucose levels, they said that the cell was in a state of internal starvation. Meanwhile, the glucose that was locked out piled up in the blood outside the cell. This is the condition we call insulin resistance.

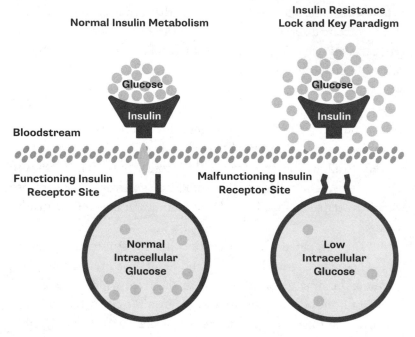

Figure 8.2. The "internal starvation" paradigm of insulin resistance

To clear the logjam, the body increases its insulin levels to "overcome" this resistance. Researchers assumed that the glucose would get shoved inside the cell by sheer brute force, lowering blood glucose levels back to normal. However, the price of normalizing blood glucose is higher blood insulin levels—hyperinsulinemia, which causes PCOS and all of the associated conditions of obesity, type 2 diabetes, cardiovascular disease, etc. Thus, insulin resistance and hyperinsulinemia are simply two sides of the same coin.

But the body only seems to be resistant to *one* of insulin's many roles: its role in glucose metabolism. The liver, for example, is not resistant to insulin in its roles in fat production or SHBG production. As insulin levels rise in the body, the liver responds by ramping up de novo lipogenesis, the process by which it converts excess dietary carbohydrates to body fat for long-term storage. In patients with insulin resistance, the liver actually appears to be *supersensitive* to insulin's effect. New fat production is significantly increased, and SHBG production in the liver is decreased.

Consider the three actions of insulin in the liver cell as follows:

1. Move glucose into cells—resistant
2. Create new fat—supersensitive
3. Decrease SHBG—supersensitive

How is it possible that the same liver cell, in response to the same glucose and insulin levels at the very same time, is both resistant and supersensitive to insulin? Insulin resistance must be selective for only certain roles. Not only that, but only certain cells show evidence of insulin resistance.

Hyperinsulinemia causes a brownish, velvety rash called acanthosis nigricans, which is often seen in the neck area. All the diseases of insulin resistance with resulting hyperinsulinemia are also associated with acanthosis nigricans. The skin cells are fully sensitive to insulin, not resistant. This seems to be another instance of selective insulin resistance.

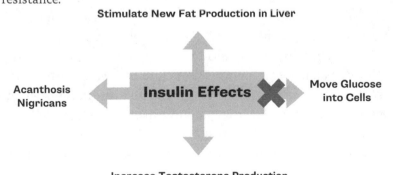

Stimulate New Fat Production in Liver

Acanthosis Nigricans

Insulin Effects

Move Glucose into Cells

Increase Testosterone Production Cystic Ovaries

Figure 8.3. Selective insulin resistance

Certain organs are resistant and certain organs are sensitive. Even within the same organ, like the liver, certain functions are resistant and others are sensitive. This idea presented a big problem for the internal starvation model of insulin resistance. If the liver cells were starved of glucose because it couldn't enter the cells during metabolism, how was the liver able to produce new fat from glucose through de novo lipogenesis? Where was the glucose coming from? Imagine trying to build a brick house without bricks. It's impossible.

Patients with hyperinsulinemic diseases, like PCOS and type 2 diabetes, were gaining fat, not losing it. With more insulin, the body continued to create fat—and that fat was being exported out of the liver as very low-density lipoprotein and taken up not only by fat cells but by the muscles, causing obesity and non-alcoholic fatty liver disease. The internal starvation paradigm was obviously incorrect. PCOS, obesity, type 2 diabetes, and fatty liver are associated with increased fat, not decreased fat, as this flawed theory predicted.

The overflow phenomenon

To understand this paradox where some actions of insulin are blocked and others are enhanced, consider another possibility. The failed internal starvation explanation supposes that something is gumming up the lock mechanism and preventing the gate from opening and admitting the glucose. But what if the opposite were true? What if the cell cannot admit glucose because *it is already overflowing*?

Let's consider an analogy. Imagine being a child packing for a trip with your parents. Your mother tells you to pack your shirts, so you take them from your closet and put them into the suitcase. Later, she finds the shirts still in the closet and, exasperated, yells at you to put the shirts in the suitcase. This is exactly what happens in cells too. Insulin tells the cells to take in glucose but finds all that glucose still in the blood. So the body releases more and more insulin, "yelling" louder and louder at the cells to move the glucose inside.

It is possible that the suitcase is locked, or the key doesn't work, or the opening mechanism is stuck—and the suitcase is empty inside.

Your mother is telling you to open up the suitcase and pack the shirts, but you cannot. This situation is analogous to the "internal starvation" model of insulin resistance: insulin is telling the cell to open up and take the glucose and it cannot.

But there's another possibility. Consider that the suitcase may already be filled with shirts. In that case, you cannot pack any more shirts in because there is no more space inside. This is the overflow condition. If the luggage is already overflowing, then yelling louder to force a few more shirts inside is not a good solution. The solution is the exact opposite: to remove some of the shirts from the luggage.

In the body, the same situation plays out. Insulin resistance, seen in PCOS, obesity, and type 2 diabetes, is an overflow situation of *too much sugar*. The liver cells are overflowing with glucose, so when insulin tells the liver to accept more glucose, it cannot. Instead, the liver is busy trying to get rid of some of the glucose by packaging it into new fat by de novo lipogenesis. This is why the liver appears to be resistant to insulin's call to move the glucose and sensitive to insulin's call to make more fat at the same time. The overflow phenomenon explains the thorny paradox of selective insulin resistance.

Since it is mainly the liver and skeletal muscles that are overfilled with glucose, there is no reason why the ovary or the skin would not react to insulin's messages. The ovary continues to make too much testosterone in response to insulin. The skin develops acanthosis nigricans in response to insulin. It is only insulin's effect on glucose that is affected because the liver and muscles are already overfilled.

THE MECHANICS OF INSULIN RESISTANCE

TO THINK ABOUT how the liver became overfilled in the first place, it is helpful to think about the luggage analogy again. The suitcase can only become overfilled if you've already been told to pack too much stuff. As the luggage fills, it is harder and harder to put more shirts in. Similarly, in the body, persistently high levels of insulin fill up the cell with glucose. As the cell fills up, it becomes more and more resistant to further calls to put more glucose inside. In other words, *too much insulin causes insulin resistance.*

If you continue to fill the overloaded suitcase, it will become harder and harder, even as your mother, thinking the suitcase is empty and underfilled, yells louder to put more shirts in. Trying to add more shirts only makes the situation worse. It's a vicious cycle. Likewise, in the body's cells, too much insulin has caused the insulin resistance. The body, "thinking" the cells are underfilled, releases more insulin to force even more glucose into an overflowing cell. This only makes the overflow situation worse. Insulin resistance causes high insulin levels—again, a vicious cycle.

In summary:

1. Too much insulin causes insulin resistance.
2. The body responds by increasing insulin levels even higher.
3. Go back to step 1.

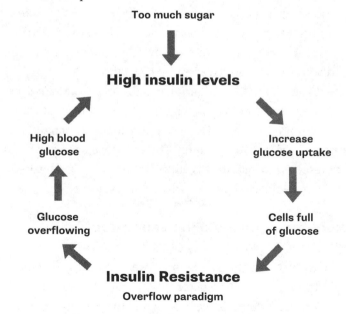

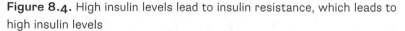

Figure 8.4. High insulin levels lead to insulin resistance, which leads to high insulin levels

Ultimately the problem is not with the suitcase. There are simply too many shirts to pack into a suitcase that can't accommodate them. In our cells, the ultimate problem is that there is too much glucose to go into cells (mostly in the liver and muscle) that cannot accommodate it. Once you understand this paradigm, the solution is simple. The packing problem has nothing to do with your mother or the suitcase. The solution is to get rid of some shirts. In the body, the problem is *too much sugar*. The solution is to either put less sugar into your body or let your body burn it off. It's a dietary solution.

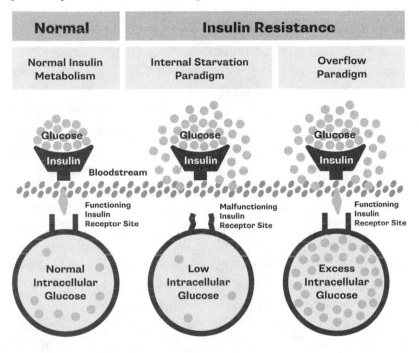

Figure 8.5. The two paradigms of insulin resistance: internal starvation versus overflow

The link between diet, insulin resistance, and PCOS

This overflow paradigm explains perfectly the selective insulin resistance seen in PCOS, type 2 diabetes, and obesity. If you eat a diet that is very high in sugar and refined carbohydrates and if you eat frequently throughout the day, you are constantly stimulating insulin, leading to hyperinsulinemia.

More glucose moves inside the cells (liver and muscles) causing overflow. The cells can't take any more glucose and have become insulin resistant. When insulin goes up yet again, the muscles and liver, already bursting, must refuse entry to glucose, which accumulates in the bloodstream.

The body, sensing this high blood glucose, responds by increasing insulin levels to "yell" at the reluctant cells to force more glucose inside. However, the intrinsic problem of overflow is not made better by this increased insulin, but *worse*. Insulin resistance increases, causing insulin to go up, causing resistance to go up. Lather. Rinse. Repeat.

Hyperinsulinemia and insulin resistance are one and the same thing viewed from different angles. They are merely two sides of the body's response to too much sugar. If you do not correct the underlying dietary problem, then the vicious cycle goes around and around, getting worse with each passing year. Insulin resistance worsens, which only drives the already high insulin levels even higher.

These high insulin levels stimulate testosterone production in the ovary and cause acne. The high insulin levels cause follicular arrest, leading to infertility, anovulatory cycles, and polycystic ovaries. The high insulin levels cause obesity and type 2 diabetes. The high insulin levels act on the skin to cause acanthosis nigricans. The high insulin levels drive the body to gain fat, causing obesity. The high insulin levels drive more new fat creation in the liver and lead to fatty liver disease. And the high insulin levels drive more insulin resistance, the disease known as type 2 diabetes.

In other words, all of the related metabolic diseases of obesity, type 2 diabetes, PCOS, and fatty liver disease are caused by the same underlying condition: too much insulin. In PCOS without type 2 diabetes, you most often find normal blood glucose levels but high blood insulin levels. This situation is often called insulin resistance. That is, insulin has succeeded in pushing glucose into the overflowing cell. But the situation has not been fixed because the moment you ease up on insulin levels, glucose will spill over again. It is a temporary Band-Aid.

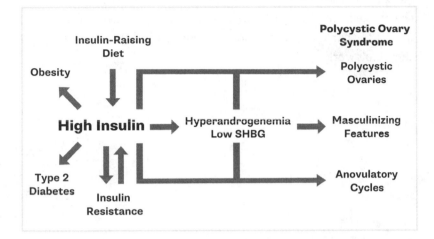

Figure 8.6. High insulin levels lead to obesity, type 2 diabetes, and PCOS

This is the key to understanding PCOS, and indeed, all of the metabolic diseases. The underlying problem is the same: *too much insulin.* The solution then becomes immediately obvious—we need to lower insulin.

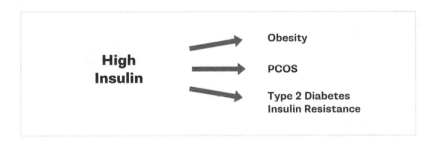

Figure 8.7. High insulin is the root cause of metabolic disease

Understanding the root cause of the problems allows us to design rational treatments. The medical treatments for PCOS should try to lower insulin since too much insulin is the root problem. Do any of the current medical therapies do this? No. That, in a nutshell, is the crux of the problem, and the reason why drugs don't work. Let's take a closer look at the current recommendations for medical treatment and why they don't work.

MELISSA

Melissa's story is not simple but it is still one of my favorites. I met Melissa in 2008 in Mozambique when she came to me for help losing weight, in the hopes that she would finally get a regular period. She had endured three unsuccessful rounds of in vitro fertilization (IVF), so conceiving a child was no longer on her radar. She and her husband, JJ, had already adopted a son named Luka and she was happy.

When I met her, Melissa had never had a regular period. She had her first period when she was 18 years old and had no more than one period a year after that. She had always been overweight, and she had some acne and male-pattern hair growth. She was soon diagnosed with PCOS. While having a baby was no longer a priority for Melissa, continually missing periods was very unhealthy and dangerous. And with PCOS, she knew she was at increased risk of developing cancer. Breast cancer ran strongly in her family, so this news was very disturbing.

After Melissa came to see me, she completely changed her diet. She cut out all refined carbs, all sugars. She lost some weight, and her periods started to come every 45 days. Knowing that Melissa wanted more children, her doctor suggested she try one more round of IVF. And success! Melissa and JJ conceived. After a healthy pregnancy, Melissa delivered Sam in May 2010. She breastfed him for two years. After that, her menstrual cycles became regular and stayed that way.

With two children, Melissa and JJ decided their family was complete. However, just a week before JJ's planned vasectomy, Melissa found out she was pregnant! She had another very healthy pregnancy and delivered another boy, Mikha, in 2013.

Today, Melissa, JJ, and their three children live in the United States. Melissa struggles a bit more with her diet there, and she notices that when she is not as strict with her carbs, her period skips a month or two. That's when Melissa knows she has to go back to her usual, strict low-carb meal plan!

PART
THREE

How Not to Treat PCOS

Medications and
Surgery

....

LIKE TO THINK that I have a pretty good understanding of PCOS, both from a professional perspective and from a personal one. I have been living with PCOS for more than 20 years, taken close to ten different medications, and undergone numerous medical procedures to mask the different expressions of this condition. I started taking the birth control pill (BCP) when I was a teenager for menstrual irregularities and acne. A few years later, my hirsutism became more apparent so I used laser hair removal, which was expensive and time-consuming. My facial hair was the worst part, because it was embarrassing and painful to remove.

In my late twenties, I stopped taking the BCP in order to start a family. After an unsuccessful year of trying to conceive naturally, I was prescribed the fertility medication clomiphene citrate, which stimulates ovulation. I could have tried in vitro fertilization (IVF), but I was uncomfortable with such an intrusive method. As a result, I was "forced" to modify my diet to see if that would work. It did, and I got pregnant.

As I mentioned earlier, though, I quickly reverted to my usual high-sugar diet and developed pre-eclampsia and high blood pressure during my pregnancy, which were treated with medications. Because my liver enzymes were elevated, a sign of impending eclampsia, my doctor performed a cesarean section. My blood pressure remained persistently high after the delivery, so I stayed on medication. Two months later, I was diagnosed with postpartum depression, for which I was prescribed yet more medication. When I tried to get pregnant with baby number two, I once again started on clomiphene, but it didn't help, so I was prescribed metformin and successfully conceived. Once again, I developed pre-eclampsia and high blood pressure and required another cesarean section.

Today I am on no medications. I am not prediabetic. I don't have high blood pressure. I am not overweight. I don't have fatty liver, acne, depression, or anxiety. I sleep well. I like how I look and how I feel. I want the same for you. But here's the secret. You cannot drug yourself to better health, because none of these drugs actually treats hyperinsulinemia, the root cause of the underlying PCOS.

Let's take a closer look at the current standard medical treatments for PCOS:

1. Symptomatic treatments
2. Fertility treatments

SYMPTOMATIC TREATMENTS

THE METHODS IN this category are prescribed to treat the wide spectrum of symptoms—from acne to excessive hair growth—that are associated with PCOS. By far the most commonly prescribed oral medication for PCOS is the birth control pill (BCP), but several other options are also available.

The birth control pill

The BCP is a hormonal contraceptive typically containing small amounts of estrogen and progestin hormones, and it has been the mainstay of drug therapy for PCOS for decades. It comes in a variety of formulations and remains one of the most widely applied treatments today. These drugs improve menstrual irregularities, reduce androgen levels, and increase liver production of sex hormone–binding globulin (SHBG),[1] which reduces symptoms such as acne and hair loss.[2] However successful at treating the symptoms, the BCP does not treat PCOS itself or its root cause (hyperinsulinemia). That is, if you stop taking the BCP, your symptoms reappear. For example, my acne returned, my coarse hairs regrew, and my menstrual irregularities resurfaced. There are also side effects to consider, including the higher risk of blood clots.[3]

Spironolactone

Spironolactone is a diuretic drug introduced in the 1960s that blocks the actions of androgens at the level of the receptor. It does not reduce androgen levels, but it blocks them from having their full effect and therefore helps alleviate symptoms such as excessive hair growth and acne.[4] Facial and body hair may be reduced by up to 40 percent with this drug.[5] Again, the symptoms will return once the drug is stopped because it does not address PCOS's underlying condition of hyperinsulinemia.

Spironolactone has several important side effects. Potassium levels frequently become elevated, sometimes to levels that can cause dangerous heart rhythms. It is also teratogenic, meaning it may cause birth defects during pregnancy. Since PCOS often affects women in their reproductive years, spironolactone must always be used with birth control to prevent pregnancy and the possibility of birth defects.[6]

Metformin

Metformin is a drug commonly prescribed in the treatment of type 2 diabetes because it improves insulin sensitivity and can thus reduce the underlying hyperinsulinemia that also causes PCOS. By 1996 the first studies showed that metformin could reduce both circulating insulin and testosterone levels. Lower insulin levels reduced ovarian production of androgens, the hallmark of PCOS.[7] Later studies confirmed that metformin could reduce circulating insulin by 35 percent, which improved every aspect of PCOS and also increased the chances of ovulation[8] and conception.

Metformin taken at least three months prior to conception increases pregnancy rates and reduces early miscarriage[9] It also lowers rates of other severe pregnancy complications, including gestational diabetes, pregnancy-induced hypertension, and pre-eclampsia, without adversely affecting the baby.[10] The American Association of Clinical Endocrinologists suggests that metformin be considered an initial therapy for women with PCOS, particularly those who are overweight or obese.[11]

Like any other drug, metformin has the potential for side effects (most often mild-to-severe gastrointestinal discomfort) but these are currently considered to be negligible compared with the drug's benefits for women with PCOS.[12]

Surgery

Surgery, like the classic ovarian wedge resection performed by Drs. Stein and Leventhal in 1935, was relatively successful[13] but is rarely used today. When all other options fail, doctors may use the less invasive laparoscopic ovarian drilling (LOD) method, which replaced ovarian wedge resection as the preferred surgical option in 1984.[14] The idea is that by surgically removing small wedges (ovarian wedge resection) of the ovary or, today, by drilling holes into the ovary (LOD), the ovary is less able to make testosterone. This reduces all the symptoms of PCOS that are caused by too much testosterone. However, the underlying problem of excess insulin is not being addressed, which exposes patients to the other metabolic effects of too much insulin—predominantly obesity and type 2 diabetes.

The complication rates from surgery are unacceptable compared with other modern medical treatments, so surgery is rarely used today. Complications include the formation of excessive scar tissue, a decrease in ovarian reserve (a woman's supply of potential eggs), and a decrease in ovarian function—all of them significant drawbacks for women wanting to conceive after surgery. Overall, LOD is not always successful, with conception rates similar to the medical (oral) therapy treatments listed above.[15]

FERTILITY TREATMENTS

BEFORE THE 1960S, treatment for anovulation consisted of psychological support, for whatever that was worth (not much). Surgery was complex and expensive, and no medications were available. In 1961 the first successful drugs were developed to promote ovulation, and the modern era of fertility medicine began.[16] Among fertility treatments, clomiphene citrate is the most common choice to start with, but again, other options are available.

Clomiphene citrate

The oral drug clomiphene citrate selectively affects estrogen receptors to stimulate ovulation. Exactly how clomiphene works is unknown, but it successfully stimulates ovulation in up to 75 to 80 percent of women and results in a live birth 20 to 50 percent of the time. The success of this drug essentially revolutionized fertility treatment, completely replacing surgery for PCOS, because it is both relatively inexpensive and highly effective.

Clomiphene does have some limitations. If it does not work in the first few months (like in my situation), it will never work and you must move on to other treatments. Combining clomiphene with other drugs such as metformin does not make it more effective. Despite these cautions, clomiphene is still considered the first-choice medication for the treatment of anovulation, underscoring exactly how little progress has been made in the understanding and treatment of this disease since the 1960s.

Letrozole

Letrozole belongs to a class of medications called aromatase inhibitors, which stimulate ovulation by preventing androgens in the body from converting into estrogen. When estrogen is blocked, the body produces follicle stimulating hormone (FSH), which stimulates the ovary to produce an egg. Compared with clomiphene citrate, letrozole produces a more physiologic hormonal stimulation that results in a lower rate of multiple births, fewer side effects, and a higher rate of live births (27.5 percent versus 19 percent).[17]

There is, however, one major concern that limits its use. Although the results are not statistically significant, some studies show a higher risk of serious birth defects.[18] Understandably, that is simply a risk that many women (and their doctors) are not willing to take.

Gonadotropins

Injectable hormones called gonadotropins can stimulate ovulation by mimicking the normal pattern of FSH and luteinizing hormone (LH), which help follicles mature and increase the chance of ovulation. The ovulation rate of women with PCOS using gonadotropins is approximately 70 percent and the pregnancy rate is approximately 20 percent.[19]

The main drawback of inducing ovulation is the risk of multiple pregnancies, with a rate as high as 10 percent. Another risk is ovarian hyperstimulation syndrome (OHSS), which can range from mild (abdominal distension and gastrointestinal discomfort such as diarrhea and nausea) to severe (enlarged ovaries, decreased urinary production, blood clots, and breathing difficulties) or even critical (death). OHSS is a potentially serious risk anytime there is ovarian stimulation, but its prevalence depends on the treatment being administered and the individual.

Intrauterine insemination and in vitro fertilization

When oral medications don't work, some women may consider more intrusive, painful, and expensive procedures for fertility, including intrauterine insemination (IUI) and IVF.

IUI is the less-invasive and less-expensive of the two procedures. A woman is given injectable gonadotropins to stimulate ovulation, and every few days, blood tests and intravaginal ultrasounds are performed to monitor the number, growth, and maturity of the follicles. Once the follicles near maturity, an injection of human chorionic gonadotropin is given to further mature the egg and promote ovulation. If ovulation occurs, a catheter with sperm (the male part of this equation) is inserted directly into the uterus to ensure that adequate sperm is available when the egg is maximally receptive. Over the next few weeks, women resume normal activities and wait for signs and symptoms of a possible pregnancy. Success rates with IUI are in the 20 percent range, slightly lower than with IVF. IUI still requires ovulation in order to be successful.

IVF is the all-in, go-for-broke treatment for fertility, where modern technology takes over as much of the baby-making process as possible. Gonadotropins are first injected to stimulate multiple egg production. Instead of relying on normal ovulation, mature eggs are retrieved surgically via ultrasound-guided needle aspiration. Sperm is combined with the eggs in a petri dish in the laboratory. Eggs successfully fertilized are transferred back into the uterus. With some luck, an embryo will implant in the wall of the uterus and develop into a growing fetus.

Women with PCOS, surprisingly, seem to have better rates of success with IVF compared with women with other fertility concerns such as tubal blockage. This is because until the age of 40 or so, women with PCOS tend to have an increased number of oocytes (immature eggs) that are amenable to being harvested for use with in vitro techniques.[20]

IVF comes with obvious physical discomfort since it involves self-injecting gonadotropins into the belly. The success rate of IVF is very difficult to measure, as it can range widely depending on a woman's health, age, reproductive history, and lifestyle, but it is estimated at between 13 and 43 percent.[21] There is a rare chance of infection associated with IVF, and as with any ovarian stimulation, the concern of OHSS. The risk of multiples (conceiving more than one fetus) is also worth considering. Some couples welcome the thought, but a multiple pregnancy comes with its own added risks, concerns, and costs. And cost is an issue for many couples. The more intrusive the treatment, the more prohibitive the cost. Each round of IVF treatment in 2005 could run to US$10,000,[22] while the estimated cost "per live birth" is much, much higher (at dozens of thousands of dollars).[23] All of these factors have a major emotional impact, and psychological concerns are common in families undergoing IVF.

As mentioned earlier in the book, Jools Oliver, a former model and the wife of celebrity chef Jamie Oliver, struggled with the symptoms of PCOS from the time she was a teenager. Her irregular periods were her most concerning problem, and when she and Jamie were unable to conceive naturally, they first resorted to clomiphene citrate and then eventually to IVF. Jools talked about experiencing dizzy spells, panic attacks, and blurred vision while undergoing IVF, to name only a few of the side effects. She and Jamie now have five children, two of whom were conceived naturally. But not everybody has the financial resources to pay for expensive IVF treatments.

A TYPICAL FERTILITY JOURNEY FOR WOMEN WITH PCOS

WOMEN WITH PCOS and obesity have a 56 percent lower chance of ovulation.[24] If you don't ovulate, you don't have any chance of getting pregnant. For women who want children and cannot get pregnant, the psychological toll can be huge, as they're unsure if they'll be able to ever have their own biological child. And with each year that passes with trying and failing to get pregnant, women hear their biological clock ticking a little louder. Many of these women will turn to fertility treatments. Here is what a typical fertility journey may look like for a woman with PCOS.

After a year of trying to spontaneously conceive, approximately 50 percent of women are unsuccessful.[25] A thorough medical workup then reveals that PCOS is the likely problem. Because the goal is to get pregnant, many of the standard medications and procedures are not used. The BCP will (obviously) prevent pregnancy. Spironolactone can cause birth defects. Metformin is generally not used during pregnancy because its safety during pregnancy is unknown. Drilling holes into the ovaries is clearly not a great boon for reproductive health. So clomiphene citrate is a typical first-choice medication, but after six months, the chance of a live birth is only about 22 percent.[26]

If the use of clomiphene fails to result in a pregnancy, doctors typically prescribe letrozole or gonadotropins. Unfortunately, these treatments also fail most of the time, and they expose women to side effects from the medications. Finally, if a woman can afford it, IUI and IVF become the only remaining medical options. Despite the expense, many people's desire to have a child is overwhelming. The outcome of IUI and/or IVF is far from certain, and the psychological and emotional roller coaster of anticipating conception and then possibly failing haunts women every month. In some cases, there is a happy ending, but others end only in tears.

Treating decreased fertility is one of the most important parts of addressing PCOS for many women, but it does not address the root cause. Yes, IVF and other fertility treatments can get you a baby, but because you still have underlying hyperinsulinemia, you have not improved your own health and you may be putting the health of your future child at risk. This point is seldom appreciated: the pregnancy of a woman with untreated PCOS is still at significantly higher risk of complications than a normal pregnancy. A pregnant woman with PCOS has an increased risk of miscarriage and maternal complications. But worse, the developing fetus is also at risk. For example, it could be large for its gestational age, which often leads to the need for a delivery by cesarean section.

There is a better solution. Instead of using drugs and other procedures to temporarily mask the symptoms of PCOS or to get pregnant—which puts both the mother and baby at risk—there is a natural solution that treats the underlying hyperinsulinemia. And that solution, as my experience and the experience of the clients I treat have shown, is diet.

Low-Calorie Diets
and Exercise

....

W HEN MY DOCTOR diagnosed me with PCOS, dietary management did not even enter into the discussion. Even though I
was lean, he expected that I would eventually become obese.
I had gained 20 to 30 pounds (9 to 14 kilograms)—an increase of 20 to
30 percent of my total body weight—in just a couple of months, so he
knew it was a BIG deal. He also knew the connection between PCOS
and obesity, and yet he assumed that I was resigned to the fact that I
would become obese. And then . . . he showed me the door. The "conver-
sation" ended there. This experience, unfortunately, is all too common
an occurrence still.

What disturbs me the most, looking back now, is that my doctor
didn't even attempt to help me address that very important factor,
weight. Obesity complicates and aggravates every aspect of PCOS. He
didn't even offer the old Eat Less, Move More option. He offered me
nothing. Instead, he focused on giving me pills, but neither medication
nor surgery reverses the underlying hyperinsulinemia at the root of
both obesity and PCOS.

Until the late 1990s, PCOS was considered mostly a disease of
excessive testosterone exposure in utero, so dietary treatment was

considered inconsequential. As the role of hyperinsulinemia and obesity became clear, however, lifestyle solutions have become, appropriately, the first-line treatment of choice. But not all diet and exercise programs are equally effective.

WHY WEIGHT LOSS IS IMPORTANT

WEIGHT LOSS IS one of the main pillars of treatment for all women with PCOS. The associated risks, such as heart disease, non-alcoholic fatty liver disease, and cancer, go up with weight gain and go down with weight loss, which cannot be said of purely symptomatic treatments like medications. Furthermore, unlike medical procedures, surgery, or medications, weight loss has practically no medically notable side effects.

Even relatively small amounts of weight loss, from 5 to 10 percent, will significantly improve all aspects of PCOS,[1] including menstrual irregularities, anovulation, and hyperandrogenism (hirsutism and acne), and improve metabolic markers such as lipids and blood sugars. Weight loss increases the likelihood that a woman will ovulate and conceive by reducing insulin levels and testosterone concentrations in the body.

Better yet, dietary interventions for fertility are very cost effective when compared with expensive medical interventions such as IVF, and they possibly offer higher rates of conception while also improving long-term health and psyche.[2] In one study, dietary modification resulted in higher rates of ovulation and conception, lower spontaneous abortion rates, and a significant cost reduction per live birth. While the cost of IVF averaged US$275,000 per live birth, the dietary program per baby cost US$4,600. Weight loss, not fertility treatments, should be considered the first option for women who are overweight and infertile.[3]

Currently, there is no consensus in the medical literature[4] about the most effective way for women with PCOS to lose that 5 to 10 percent of body weight, and thus most women are guided toward the standard dietary advice to count their calories and increase their exercise. This approach, known as Eat Less, Move More—or sometimes Calories In, Calories Out—is where all the trouble begins. As we saw in chapter 4, measuring calories is ineffective. This standard Eat Less, Move More advice is clear, simple, and *almost completely ineffective.*

Advertising and the popularity of the low-calorie myth

Most diets today focus on caloric restriction rather than dietary composition.[5] This approach, known as the Calories In, Calories Out approach, is familiar to most people. It assumes that the fattening effect of a food is solely a reflection of its caloric content. In other words, a calorie is a calorie. Since dietary fat is higher in calories per gram than either carbohydrates or protein, the most efficient method of cutting calories is to reduce dietary fat by adopting a low-fat diet.

Despite ample evidence that shows 200 calories of cookies are not equal to 200 calories of salmon, as a society we still believe that calories are the most important determinant of weight gain. Why do we believe so strongly in this calorie myth? Because of advertising, that's why. Snack food manufacturers have spent millions of dollars convincing us that all calories are equally fattening. Cookie makers do not want you to believe that cookies are more fattening than beef. Candy makers do not want you to know that candy is more fattening than spinach. No, that's no way to sell cookies and candy. They would rather have you believe that cookies and salmon are equally fattening as long as the calories are equal. And believe me, I can tell you all about eating cookies for dinner and candy, candy, candy all the time. That's pretty much how I developed PCOS.

Soda companies heavily promote the Calories In, Calories Out model because they desperately need you (the consumer) to believe that it is not sugar that is making you fat, but calories. The simple, obvious truth that sugar and refined grains make you fat would devastate the companies' profits. So they give millions of dollars to "researchers" who are willing to promote that view.[6] In 2016, in response to growing criticisms about transparency, Coca-Cola released a list of organizations, including researchers, who took their money.[7] Chump change? Hardly.

In 2015 Coca-Cola gave millions of dollars to doctors at the University of Colorado to set up a nonprofit organization called the Global Energy Balance Network.[8] According to the *New York Times*, Dr. Hill, the nonprofit's president, also proposed a study to "help Coca-Cola focus the blame for obesity on a lack of exercise and urged the company to pay for it."[9] Coke carefully hid its name behind the university, and the doctors were well-paid for their part. Once these shenanigans were revealed by the *New York Times*, Dr. Willett of Harvard University accused the group of spreading "scientific nonsense." Of course it was nonsense. But it was lucrative nonsense. The Global Energy Balance Network no longer exists. It discontinued operations in 2015 after the *New York Times* article appeared, and the $1 million the organization had received was refunded to Coca-Cola.

The first step in deflecting blame is to find the appropriate scapegoat. In the case of sugar causing obesity, calories make the perfect scapegoat. There is no brand called Calories. Nobody owns the trademark Calories. Nobody makes food called Calories. Calories deflect attention from sugar. But this is ridiculous: claiming that all calories are equal is just like claiming that all drugs are equal. And the same number of milligrams of deadly cyanide and of Aspirin—no matter how big or small—is not going to have the same effect. That is not the question we asked. We never asked if a drug is a drug. We want to know if all drugs are equally toxic. Similarly, we never asked if a calorie is a calorie. We want to know if all calories are equally fattening. The simple and obvious reality is that drugs differ greatly in their effect on the human body. Similarly, candy and kale have utterly different metabolic effects on the human body and weight.

Focusing on calories is a trap, pure and simple. Obesity is a *hormonal*, not a caloric imbalance. Thus, you must adjust the hormones in order to lose weight. Insulin is the main driver of both obesity and PCOS, so the solution is to lower insulin. Why, then, do doctors continue to prescribe low-fat diets for weight loss?

Clinical inertia in the medical community

The low-fat, calorie-restricted diet has been used for many decades with spectacular failure for weight loss. If firsthand evidence wasn't enough to prove this, the Women's Health Initiative (WHI),[10] the largest and most important nutrition study ever done, certainly has. Almost 50,000 women were randomized into the trial and given instructions to reduce their fat intake. Over seven years, women reduced their calorie intake by 361 calories per day. They reduced their percentage of calories from fat and increased their carbs. They also increased their daily exercise by 10 percent. When the results were published in 2006, they showed that women who cut their calories did not lose much weight, did not have slimmer waists, and did not have any cardiovascular benefits compared with women who simply continued to eat as they had before.

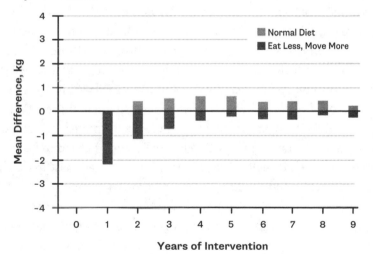

Figure 10.1. Minimal weight loss using the Eat Less, Move More dietary strategy[11]

Interestingly, the WHI proved conclusively what almost every dieter in the world already knows. Cutting calories doesn't result in long-term weight loss. Women who cut their calories lost weight at first, but over the first year their weight plateaued and then crept back up to their original weight. And this happened *even though women continued to follow their diet*! Every study done of calorie restriction shows the exact same results. Yet, illogically, medical professionals and nutritional authorities continue to recommend this diet for the control of obesity and PCOS.

Some physicians play the blame game, insisting that their scientifically unproven caloric-reduction advice is flawless, but that their patients are not following these low-calorie diets properly. In other words, it isn't *their* fault you aren't losing weight. It's *yours*. Others simply ignore the science, preferring to keep their preconceived notions rather than devising more robust alternative theories. Unfortunately, many medical practitioners seem to have taken this approach and the ground-breaking WHI study has largely been ignored and relegated to the dustbins of nutritional history.

Despite the fact that many in the medical community are willfully blind to the evidence, we know that calorie consumption is under tight hormonal control. Weight loss leads to persistent elevations in ghrelin (a hormone), which leads to increased hunger even a year after weight loss. Patients on calorie-reduced diets who regained weight after a year did not lose their willpower; they were measurably hungrier. Calorie-reduced diets fail over the long term because hormones regulate our basal metabolic rate—the baseline level of energy needed to keep our bodies running normally. Low caloric intake reduces basal metabolic rates as much as 40 percent in an effort to conserve energy.[12]

Fat accumulation is really not a problem of energy excess. It's a problem of energy *distribution*. Our hormones decide how that energy is used. For example, we cannot decide how much energy to expend on accumulating fat versus forming new bone or increasing body temperature. Different foods evoke different hormonal responses.

Remember, 200 calories of cookies will metabolize very differently than 200 calories of salmon. Therefore, the important thing is how to control the hormonal signals we receive from food, not the total number of calories we eat.

Similarly, moving more—while it improves psychosocial parameters, self-esteem, muscle mass, and bone mass—will not automatically lead to weight loss, nor will it resolve the root cause of PCOS.

WHY EXERCISE ALONE IS NOT THE SOLUTION

I MET ANDREA, now an excellent personal trainer, back in my university days. She was fit! That's my best description of her. She tried her best to help me get fit, but to no avail. Andrea, although not thin, was super-muscular and occasionally competed in body building. Interestingly, Andrea's dietary habits were very similar to mine. We ate many times per day and ate lots of carbohydrate-rich foods, although she also added some extra protein shakes (probably more often than I can recall). Andrea was trying to "fuel" her workouts, and there was a big push in athletic circles for "carb-loading" regimens.

Andrea and I stayed in touch while I was in Mozambique, and when I returned to Canada ten years later, I reconnected with her. We both looked different. I had gained some weight (I was short, chubby, and pregnant) and Andrea was still fit but had grown a "belly." No matter how hard she tried "cutting calories" and exercising more, she still couldn't get rid of that belly. As we shared our common fertility struggles, I learned that we had both been diagnosed with PCOS. Andrea and her husband had never become pregnant, though, and were looking into adoption.

Obviously I told her every detail of my own journey to get pregnant, and Andrea became my "patient." As I counseled her, I created a website to share recipes and information about low-carb diets, fertility, and eventually intermittent fasting. We started by eliminating "sugars" from her diet and then gradually replaced the other "carbier" foods with nonstarchy vegetables containing more fiber and with healthier sources of fat such as avocados, eggs, and olive oil. She soon felt more "satisfied" and less need to snack between meals. Within months, she adopted a schedule of intermittent fasting known as time-restricted eating, in which she ate two meals per day but only during a six-hour period. For the other 18 hours, she fasted. Some days Andrea ate at 8 a.m. and 2 p.m., other days at 12 p.m. and 6 p.m., depending on her workout schedule. She soon reported that she felt stronger than ever and her workouts had improved!

From years of dieting and working as a personal trainer, Andrea was used to counting calories. She was surprised to find that her caloric intake actually *increased* on this low-carbohydrate, high–healthy fat diet, yet not only did she lose that darn belly, she gained another one... I think you know how this story ends: Andrea had a baby girl at 39 years old and a baby boy at 41.

So is Andrea's story evidence that exercise is not the answer? We know the root cause of PCOS is hyperinsulinemia, which causes the polycystic ovaries to overproduce androgens, and that to treat this disease we need to lower insulin. What role, if any, does exercise play in reversing PCOS?

The relationship between exercise and PCOS

Women with PCOS are more insulin resistant and have more visceral (belly) fat than the general population, and exercise can help reduce both. Further, it may lower triglycerides[13] and inflammatory markers like hs-CRP (high-sensitivity C-reactive protein), both risk factors for heart disease.[14] Given the benefits of moderate exercise in lowering insulin resistance, it seems natural that exercise be an integral part of lifestyle changes for PCOS. However, only five small studies have looked at the effects of exercise on PCOS.[15] Only three of those five studies showed that exercise contributes to an improvement in menstrual symptoms. Only one study measured the effect of exercise on how quickly women get pregnant, and it was inconclusive.

Part of the problem with studies of exercise intervention is the high dropout rate. Usually 30 to 50 percent of participants in the exercise group dropped out, and longer-duration studies had higher dropout rates. The most successful studies involved supervised exercise regimens of moderate intensity, three times per week.

Another limitation is that no specific guidelines exist for exercise in relation to PCOS. In 2008 the U.S. Department of Health and Human Services suggested 150 minutes of moderate-intensity activity per week for women with PCOS, so this amount of exercise falls within the general purview of what is recommended for all adults.[16] Approximately 60 percent of women with PCOS also meet this goal.

Despite the lack of research into exercise and PCOS specifically, the failure of exercise to cause significant weight loss is well-known in research, and the reason for failure is called compensation. People who increase their exercise will likely

1. eat more (increase caloric intake) and
2. decrease activity outside of the prescribed exercise.

These compensatory responses reduce the effectiveness of exercise as a weight-loss tool.[17] The main reason for the failure of exercise, though, is that it fails to address the root cause of both obesity and PCOS—hyperinsulinemia. Obesity and PCOS are conditions caused by too much insulin, not by too little exercise. Increased exercise may reduce insulin, but only mildly, and is thus a very inefficient method of treating the hyperinsulinemia. Therefore, exercise without dietary changes is not a great weight-loss tool.[18] And there is no solid evidence, clinical or otherwise, that exercise alone can reverse PCOS.[19] In other words, you can't outrun a bad diet!

Professor Tim Noakes knows that all too well. He is a physician, researcher, and emeritus professor recognized for his large body of work and research in exercise physiology and for his numerous books, including the classic *Lore of Running* that touted the benefits of a high-carbohydrate diet for runners. He has run more than 70 marathons and ultramarathons, yet despite all this exercise he found himself battling weight gain and type 2 diabetes caused largely by a diet high in sugar and refined carbohydrates. More recently, however, his view of the primary role of nutrition in obesity has changed and he's been quoted as saying, "If you've got *Lore of Running*, tear out the section on nutrition." His (and coauthors') 2015 bestseller *The Real Meal Revolution* suggests that a low-carbohydrate diet of real food may reverse the obesity epidemic not only in his home country of South Africa but also around the world. These ideas have been controversial: at one point, he had to defend his views in a three-year trial brought forth by the Health Professions Council of South Africa, which threatened to revoke his medical license.

Obesity is clearly linked to polycystic ovary syndrome (PCOS), so changes in the treatment of obesity have crucial implications for PCOS too. Insulin is a nutrient sensor that goes up when we eat. Too much insulin over too long a period of time leads to insulin resistance, particularly in the liver. No matter how much exercise you do, you cannot reduce insulin unless you change your diet. If you eat, insulin goes up. If you eat and exercise, insulin goes up. There is no change to the underlying problem of obesity and PCOS. Further, the liver is the key player in the development of insulin resistance. You cannot exercise your liver.

Neither does exercise alone seem to improve fertility rates. Even in studies that showed improved ovulation rates, there was no significant increase in pregnancy rates.[20] The benefit, albeit small, is likely due to the small indirect effect of improved insulin resistance. This seems to be supported by what other researchers have found.[21] Although weight loss via diet improved reproductive function, adding exercise did not. What it did do was improve body composition (reduction in central obesity).

Exercise and insulin are largely independent factors. There may be a small indirect effect of exercise improving insulin resistance in the skeletal muscles, so it is not entirely useless. However, exercise is also not particularly useful in reducing the effects of PCOS.

VERONICA

Veronica had just turned 41. She, along with her husband, Z, had been trying to conceive for over a year. They had tried intrauterine inseminations twice but those were not successful. And Veronica had had two miscarriages. Although she was never diagnosed with PCOS, I believed that dietary changes would significantly improve her fertility. I knew that, given she was in her forties, she felt pressure to conceive quickly, just as I knew that because she was older, she was more likely to have metabolic syndrome (i.e., obesity, diabetes, and hypertension). Lowering insulin helps everyone, but especially older women and those with metabolic syndrome.

Just one month after starting a low-carb diet and intermittent fasting, Veronica and Z successfully conceived. Although Veronica did not stick to a strict low-carb diet during her pregnancy, she had no gestational diabetes or pre-eclampsia and she delivered a beautiful, healthy baby girl. She did, however, jump back into a low-carb diet with more intermittent fasting to help her lose the pregnancy weight (which she did).

PART
FOUR

How to Effectively
Treat PCOS

The Optimal Diet
for PCOS

....

F YOU SUFFER from PCOS, then you need to follow an insulin-lowering diet, which is not necessarily low in calories. You need to know what foods have a high or low insulin effect. You also need to know when to eat those foods. The optimal diet for PCOS has two parts: what to eat and when to eat.

WHAT TO EAT
....

ALL CARBOHYDRATES WILL produce an insulin response, but the biggest culprit is the refined carbohydrates such as sweets, white bread, and flour. Unprocessed carbohydrates, such as legumes and tubers, have much lower insulin stimulation compared with processed carbohydrates such as bread and sugar. The standard low-fat, calorie-reduced diet is typically high in carbohydrates because it follows the original 1977 U.S. dietary guidelines, which suggested carbohydrates constitute 55 to 60 percent of the diet. This amount might be OK if we were eating a lot of sweet potatoes like the Okinawans, but we were directed to eat 6–11 servings per day of highly refined grains in the bread, cereal, rice, and pasta group, which will raise insulin tremendously.

Refined carbohydrates generate the largest insulin response; dietary protein, particularly animal protein, also has a significant insulin response; and dietary fat, almost none at all. Protein, however, has the greatest effect on satiety, which makes us feel full. Thus, the optimal diet for reducing insulin limits refined carbohydrates, because the body does not need carbohydrates for good health, and it includes a moderate amount of dietary protein, since we need a certain amount to maintain health. But because it can also cause a significant insulin response and because the body cannot store excess dietary protein, eating more than is needed is not recommended. Dietary fat, on the other hand, should not be feared and should be included. This may come as a bit of a shock if you've lived through the fat phobia of the 1980s and 1990s.

Need proof? The brilliant Cambridge-educated researcher Dr. Zoë Harcombe demonstrated there is no evidence that dietary fat contributes in a meaningful way to the development of heart disease.[1] (She is my female crush, by the way!) In her fascinating book *The Big Fat Surprise: Why Butter, Meat, and Cheese Belong in a Healthy Diet*, the American journalist and author Nina Teicholz details the roots of our epic misunderstanding about dietary fat. And the largest nutritional trial ever done, the Women's Health Initiative (WHI), also proved that reducing dietary fat does not reduce cardiovascular disease.[2] It showed that eating a low-fat diet carries the same risk of heart disease as a higher-fat diet. It is on the back of studies such as the WHI's that the term "healthy fat" has gradually entered the lexicon, as we've started to realize that eating fat is not going to kill us.

Introducing my low-carb diet

Today's low-carbohydrate diets typically allow less than 50 grams of carbohydrates per day (compared with 100 to 200 grams in the 1970s and 1980s). The diet I recommend—a very low-carbohydrate, moderate-protein, high–healthy fat diet—restricts carbohydrates to less than 20 grams per day.

Restricting dietary carbohydrates to 20 grams per day puts glucose in limited supply. Remember that glucose is the body's short-term source of energy. Most of the body can access the long-term energy stores by metabolizing fat, but the brain cannot. Fat does not pass through the blood-brain barrier. To supply energy for the brain when glucose is scarce, the liver metabolizes fat (either dietary fat or body fat) and produces ketone bodies. The word "ketogenic" comes from the body's production of these ketone bodies, a natural process called ketosis. It should not be confused with ketoacidosis, a pathological situation that occurs in type 1 diabetics when the body does not have enough insulin to obtain the energy it needs.

Ketosis triggered via a low-carbohydrate diet is not intrinsically harmful in the long term. Children with intractable seizures have been successfully treated by eating a low-carb diet, which they must maintain for their entire lives to stay free of the seizures. Studies show their health is otherwise completely normal on this long-term high-fat diet; there is no evidence of excessive heart disease.[3] There is no reason to fear eating dietary fat: it does not make you fat and does not cause heart disease. Enjoy lots of natural fats, such as olive oil, nuts, and avocados, but stay away from highly inflammatory, highly processed fats such as vegetable oils.

Although the terms "ketogenic diet" and "keto diet" are in common use, and the low-carb diet I describe in this book *is* a strict ketogenic diet, I prefer to call my recommended diet simply a low-carb diet. My intent is not to raise ketones, but rather to lower insulin. The increase of ketones is simply a result of lowering insulin. As with any eating regimen that gains popularity, there will be companies and others that use the keto terminology incorrectly. When looking for recipes, keep this in mind and follow the basic principles of the low-carb diet: low carbohydrates, moderate protein, high healthy fats.

An optimal insulin-lowering diet consists of the following steps:
1. Severely restrict added sugars.
2. Severely restrict refined carbohydrates, particularly grains.
3. Moderate intake of dietary protein.
4. Eat natural fats liberally.

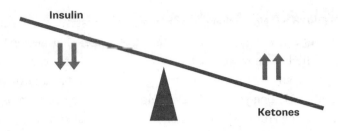

Figure 11.1. Insulin versus ketones: a seesaw inverse correlation

WHEN TO EAT

EATING, BY ITS very nature, raises insulin. The mixture of carbohydrate, fat, and protein in the food determines to what degree. Eating continually keeps your insulin levels high. In contrast, not eating, called fasting, allows your insulin to fall. Eating raises insulin and fasting drops insulin. Thus, to lower insulin levels to treat PCOS, simply spend more time fasting and less time eating.

Skip the snacks (and kick your cravings too)

Prior to 1977, not only did we eat more dietary fat and fewer refined grains, we also ate less often. There were no official recommendations to change our eating patterns but we did, and I believe this contributed equally to the obesity crisis. The National Health and Nutrition Examination Survey (NHANES) study[4] in 1977 found that most people ate three times per day: breakfast, lunch, and dinner. If you wanted an after-school snack, your mom said, "No, you'll ruin your dinner." If you wanted a bedtime snack, she just said no. Snacking was considered neither necessary nor healthy. A snack was a treat, to be taken only very occasionally. Yet now, we are often told that eating more frequently will help weight loss. No scientific data supports this assumption, and it has gained respectability only through mindless repetition. At first glance, it sounds pretty stupid. And it sounds stupid because it is stupid.

The Adventist Health Study 2 looked at the dietary habits of over 50,000 adults and found that the more often they ate, the heavier they were likely to be.[5] Not rocket science. If you eat constantly, you will gain more weight. The study also noted that the longer that people fasted at night, the less they weighed. Again, not really hard to understand. If you give your body more time to digest your food and burn stored food (body fat), then you will likely weigh less. But by 2004, most people were eating almost six times per day. It is almost considered abuse to deprive your child of a mid-morning or after-school snack or a juice-and-cookie pick-me-up at half time in their sports game. And we wonder why we have a childhood obesity crisis! Why did we change our ways?

The reason is most likely related to heavy advertising by food companies. No scientific study has ever proven that snacking causes weight loss or is even healthy. But that's the power of advertising. Without any science to back it up, many nutritional authorities have now endorsed eating multiple times per day as a healthy practice. There really is no such thing as a healthy snack. Recent studies show that fewer than 10 percent of people eat three times per day or less.[6] And 10 percent of people ate an astounding 10 times per day. Essentially, many people start eating as soon as they get up and don't stop until they go to bed. The median time during which people eat is 14.75 hours per day; that is, if they break their fast at 8 a.m., they don't, on average, put the last bite of food in their mouth until 10:45 p.m.! Practically the only time people stopped eating was while sleeping. This contrasts with a 1970s-era style of eating the first meal, breakfast, at 8 a.m. and the last meal, dinner, at 6 p.m., an eating duration of only 10 hours.

By reducing snacks, we allow our body the time it needs to digest food from a meal and metabolize it before putting more food into our mouths. One further problem with snacks is that they need to be relatively easy to carry (portable) and convenient, requiring little cooking. Snack foods are often highly processed and prepackaged, containing refined grains and sugar, which do not require refrigeration. After all, very few people will grill a small piece of salmon for a mid-morning snack.

Many people have trouble giving up snacks because of food cravings—those frequent, intense urges to eat sugary foods, or salty foods, or carbohydrate-rich foods, or chocolate, or "junk" foods. Even though we know intellectually that these foods will make us gain weight, we feel helpless to resist them. It's like an itch we have to scratch. But there's also a lot of misinformation about why we crave foods, and these are used to support snacking. So let's debunk them.

Myth #1. Food cravings develop in response to deficiencies of certain nutrients. This idea is clearly not true. The most common foods people crave, such as sweets or potato chips, contain no essential nutrients. Soda has no essential nutrients. Doughnuts have no essential nutrients. So what nutrients are we talking about?

Myth #2. Food cravings develop in the absence of food. One of the persistent myths about fasting is that you'll get so hungry that you will be forced to stuff your face with Krispy Kreme doughnuts, which is why people recommend that you eat six or seven times a day—to stave off those cravings. These people obviously don't have any practical experience with fasting, and don't understand the research, which shows exactly the opposite. If you eat constantly, you are more likely to feed those cravings. If you eat less often, you not only reduce your food cravings, you also reduce your feelings of hunger. Research shows that severe caloric restriction was much, much more effective at reducing cravings than a higher-calorie (1200 kilocalories/day) diet.[7] In my experience and in the literature,[8] fasting when done consistently decreases hunger.

It is possible that the consistent association of certain foods with particular stimuli or social contexts may lead to cravings. For example, cake and special occasions. Doughnuts and coffee breaks. The research shows that abstinence will diminish those cravings. Like an itch, giving in to a craving only makes it worse. The solution is to stop scratching an itch, to kick the habit. Eating very little or nothing (as in fasting) has the potential to completely eliminate cravings. Eating a moderately restricted diet has virtually no effect on cravings. People who reduce their sugar intake very close to zero, for example, find that their sweet tooth goes away. In contrast, if you eat more sugar, cravings don't get better—they get worse.

That's great news, because now you are working with your body to lose weight instead of working against it.

Eat earlier in the day

The exact same food will elicit different insulin responses at different times of the day. Studies show that the same meal taken at dinner, compared with breakfast, produces almost 30 percent more insulin effect.[9] Food is more fattening when you eat it later at night because more of the food energy (calories) is directed toward storage rather than usage.

The body's circadian rhythm—the natural, internal system that regulates feelings of sleepiness and wakefulness—also affects appetite. Hunger is lowest in the morning and greatest in the evening, around 8 p.m. or so.[10] Other studies show that eating later at night results in a lower metabolic rate.[11] If your metabolism is burning fewer calories, weight loss is harder.

So eating your largest meal late in the day gives you three problems:

1. You'll eat more (because you are hungrier—yikes).
2. The food you eat is more fattening (because it raises insulin levels higher—double yikes).
3. You'll expend less energy (and more calories will get turned to fat—triple yikes).

We tend to eat later only because of our work-life schedules, not because it is healthy. Since many people work or go to school during the day, we leave our main meal, which we eat as a family, until the evening. And this dinner often gets pushed later and later into the evening because of longer commuting times and more families in which both parents work outside the home. But understand that habitually eating later increases the insulin and, therefore, the fattening effect of food.

Fast intermittently (using a time-restricted eating strategy)

Skipping snacks is a great start for lowering your insulin levels, but you can go further by integrating some intermittent fasting. This sounds really scary, but fasting is simply defined as any period of time that you are not eating. Generally, people should be fasting for a minimum of 12 hours per night. For example, if you eat dinner at 8 p.m. and breakfast at 8 a.m., that is a 12-hour fasting period. Remember, breakfast, no matter what time it happens, is the meal that breaks your fast.

There are an infinite number of ways to fast. They generally differ by the length of time during which you don't eat and the liquids you're allowed to drink during the fast. You can fast for 12 hours, 16 hours, 24 hours, 36 hours, 42 hours, or multiple days. During a classic fast, only water is allowed. However, you can still obtain good results by allowing other fluids, including tea, herbal tea, coffee, and bone broth. And that's what I recommend you do.

The cardinal rule of fasting, or indeed of any kind of dietary change, is to always make sure you are doing it safely. In the past, fasting often meant going for days or weeks without food. That's not what I'm suggesting here. Longer fasts have more power but more risk, and there is no reason to fast for five consecutive days just for the sake of doing it. Intermittent fasting means fasting consistently and frequently for shorter periods of time. In other words, why not do five separate 24-hour fasts over a number of weeks or months instead? This approach will have roughly the same beneficial health effects with far less risk. One of the easiest forms of intermittent fasting is called time-restricted eating. It can be as simple as fasting for 16 hours of the day and eating within an eight-hour window.

Before you begin any fast, consult your doctor, especially if you are diabetic or taking medications. Intermittent fasting is entirely safe for most people, but you should not fast for more than 16 to 18 hours at a time if you are

1. underweight or malnourished (Body Mass Index or BMI under 20),[12]
2. pregnant or breastfeeding, or
3. under the age of 18.

During the fasting period, the body must survive on its stored nutrients and food energy. If you do not have lots of body fat (stored food energy), then your body will not be able to function properly, which will put your health at risk. Similarly, extended fasting is also not recommended during pregnancy or breastfeeding or for children under 18. A fetus, baby, or child needs adequate nutrition to grow, and deliberately limiting nutrients risks the chance of permanent damage.

Always make sure that you feel well during the fast. You may feel hungry, maybe a little irritable, constipated perhaps, but you should not feel *unwell*. If you are really feeling poorly, break your fast. For example, if you feel extremely weak or unable to get out of bed, then there is something wrong and you should stop fasting immediately. Fasting is free! You will not lose money. You will not lose out on the chance to try again. Electrolyte depletion, especially sodium and magnesium, is common. Don't push beyond the limits of safety and common sense. It is far better to stop and, if you want, begin again in a few days when you are feeling better.

Fasting, done properly and with knowledge and experience, is a powerful tool in the fight against obesity, metabolic disease, and PCOS. Fasting used inappropriately can hurt or kill you. So learn to use this tool properly. Don't dive right into a 30-day water-only fast. Instead, begin by skipping a meal here and there.

Intermittent diets work better than constant ones. Just as walking from a dark room into daylight is often blinding until your eyes adjust after several minutes, fasting jolts our bodies out of their established dieting patterns. The MATADOR study[13] randomized patients to either a block of constant dieting or a two-week period of dieting alternating with a two-week period of no energy restriction. Both groups got eight weeks of dieting, but one group was constant and the other intermittent. The difference in weight loss at six months was astounding: people in the intermittent fasting group had lost 13.6 pounds—6.2 kilograms—more! A separate study[14] found that patients who ate only between 8 a.m. and 2 p.m.—that is, an intermittent fasting strategy of a daily 18-hour fast with food taken early in the day—had lower insulin, insulin resistance, and blood pressure than before they began.

Among the other important lessons learned in that study is that there is an adaptation period to time-restricted eating.[15] It took participants 12 days, on average, to adjust, so don't give up on it after just a couple of days: it can take up to three or four weeks for some people to adjust. Most people found the fasting period relatively easy to adhere to—it's not hard to fast for 16 or 18 hours—but they found it more difficult to adjust to the time restriction. Eating dinner at 2 p.m. is tough for people who work or go to school during the day. An interesting finding was that people who restricted late-night eating had less desire to eat and also less capacity to eat. They couldn't eat more at night even if they wanted to! It is obviously easier to restrict eating if you are not hungry, and some of that benefit may be due to reductions in food cravings.

Overall, then, the most effective dietary strategy to combat PCOS is to combine all these principles:

1. Don't snack, "graze," or give in to food cravings.
2. Eat your meals early in the day.
3. Fast intermittently using a time-restricted eating strategy.

Now that we've established generally what to eat to prevent and reverse PCOS and when to eat it, let's get more specific so we can start cooking!

Practical Advice
and Recipes for
Women with PCOS

....

I HAVE READ HUNDREDS of scientific articles, books, blogs, and websites that purport to help women with PCOS. All agree that weight loss through diet and lifestyle are important. But their recommended diet of eating frequent low-fat, low-calorie meals achieves just the opposite. Similarly, many of my patients tell me that they have tried every diet out there and the results are always the same: initially they lose some weight and eventually they gain all that weight back.

But let me share with you another story, a success story. I met Maria José over 20 years ago when I worked part-time at a bank while attending university. She was my supervisor. Fifteen years later, she became my client when I attended naturopathic college, and I have followed her weight journey ever since. At the beginning of my career, I advised "Ze" to follow a lower-calorie diet because that's all I knew. You can guess the result: she lost 100 pounds (45 kilograms) and then gained it back. When I left for Mozambique right after naturopathic college, Ze tried many other diets—she juiced, she drank protein shakes, she took weight-loss supplements—all with the same result. The definition of insanity is doing the same thing over and over again and expecting different results. Ze felt "insane."

When I returned from Mozambique, she knew that I was following a very different approach and she became my client once again in the fall of 2016. By that time, I knew about PCOS, and though Ze never received an official diagnosis, she showed all the signs. We started by cutting out snacks and grazing while she continued to eat three full meals per day. In the first month, she lost 5.5 pounds (2.5 kilograms). In the second month, we introduced 18-hour intermittent fasts. She started to eat two meals per day and we began to reduce her carbs and introduce more healthy fats to her diet. Ze felt satisfied and satiated between meals and she lost 8.8 pounds (4 kilograms) that month. Christmas came along and she enjoyed holiday meals with her friends and family, which led her to gain just over a pound (half a kilogram). In January, she got back to her low-carbohydrate diet, began fasting for 24 hours on alternate days, and quickly lost 5.5 pounds (2.5 kilograms).

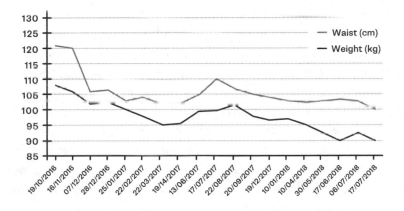

Figure 12.1. Maria José's Intensive Dietary Management chart: weight and waist measurements from October 2016 to July 2018

In 18 months, Ze lost a total of 40.8 pounds (18.5 kilograms). The best part is that she's committed to this lifestyle. Even with extended visits to her family in Costa Rica and a vacation in Cuba, Ze has lost

8.5 inches (21 centimeters) from around her waist—more than ever before. That's because this is not a "diet." This lifestyle approach addresses her insulin resistance, and not her caloric intake! I'm already very proud of her.

Here are the practical steps you need to take to reduce insulin and lose weight. Follow these guidelines and you'll be well on your way to managing PCOS and overcoming infertility—naturally.

ELIMINATE ADDED SUGARS

SUGAR STIMULATES INSULIN but is also uniquely fattening because it directly produces insulin resistance.

Cut out sugar-sweetened beverages. One of the biggest dietary sources of sugar is found in drinks. If you haven't already, eliminate the sugar from your teas and coffees, including iced teas and iced coffees or cappuccinos. Stop drinking fruit juices, soda pop, smoothies, slushies, and sport drinks—all of which are full of sugar. Although lemonade does not always taste sweet, it is. Cut it from your diet too.

Eliminate processed and prepared foods. Added sugars, the ones added in processing and manufacturing, are more dangerous than naturally occurring sugars for several reasons. First, they may be added in unlimited amounts. Second, they may be found in much higher concentrations. For example, candy is virtually 100 percent sugar, whereas even the sweetest fruits do not contain that much sugar. Third, they contain no dietary fiber to offset the harmful effects. That is, I can eat three or more bags of candy (it has happened) but I can never finish a bag of fruit. For these reasons, direct your efforts toward reducing added sugars as opposed to naturally occurring sugars.

Added sugar goes by a lot of different names, including sucrose, glucose, fructose, maltose, dextrose, molasses, hydrolyzed starch, honey, invert sugar, cane sugar, glucose-fructose, high-fructose corn syrup, brown sugar, corn sweetener, rice/corn/cane/maple/malt/golden/palm syrup, and agave nectar.

Food labels list ingredients in order of how much is contained, so if you can break up the added sugar into different ingredients, such as sugar, brown sugar, and corn syrup, then sugar will not be the first ingredient. Watch for this trick; here's an example from a breakfast cereal.

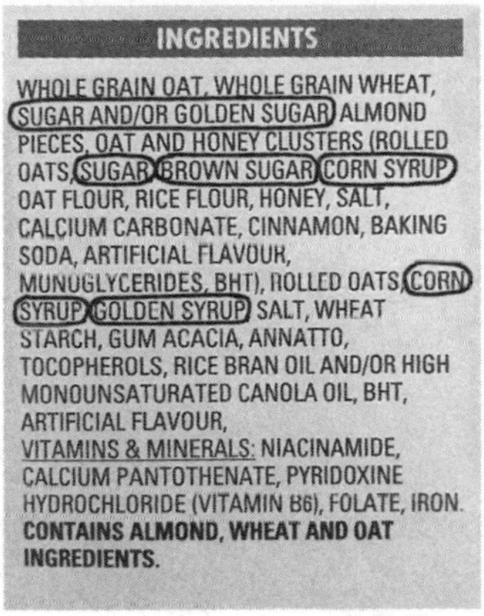

INGREDIENTS

WHOLE GRAIN OAT, WHOLE GRAIN WHEAT, SUGAR AND/OR GOLDEN SUGAR, ALMOND PIECES, OAT AND HONEY CLUSTERS (ROLLED OATS, SUGAR, BROWN SUGAR, CORN SYRUP, OAT FLOUR, RICE FLOUR, HONEY, SALT, CALCIUM CARBONATE, CINNAMON, BAKING SODA, ARTIFICIAL FLAVOUR, MONOGLYCERIDES, BHT), ROLLED OATS, CORN SYRUP, GOLDEN SYRUP, SALT, WHEAT STARCH, GUM ACACIA, ANNATTO, TOCOPHEROLS, RICE BRAN OIL AND/OR HIGH MONOUNSATURATED CANOLA OIL, BHT, ARTIFICIAL FLAVOUR, VITAMINS & MINERALS: NIACINAMIDE, CALCIUM PANTOTHENATE, PYRIDOXINE HYDROCHLORIDE (VITAMIN B6), FOLATE, IRON. **CONTAINS ALMOND, WHEAT AND OAT INGREDIENTS.**

Figure 12.2. The many names of sugar

Sugar adds flavor to processed foods at virtually no cost (to the manufacturer). Pay particular attention to sauces, such as barbecue, plum, honey-garlic, hoisin, sweet and sour, and other dipping sauces. Spaghetti sauce, too, can contain as much as 10 to 15 grams (3 to 4 teaspoons) of sugar per serving. Commercial salad dressings and condiments, such as ketchup and relish, also often contain lots of sugar. The bottom line is this: if it comes in a package, then it likely contains added sugar.

Ideally, avoid these products altogether or buy the version with the least amount of added sugars.

Avoid foods and beverages made with artificial sweeteners. Artificial sweeteners, such as aspartame, sucralose, or acesulfame-K, raise insulin as much as sugar and are equally prone to causing obesity. Sweeteners give a false promise of sweetness without consequence. Between 1960 and 2000, the use of diet drinks rocketed;[1] however, the obesity and diabetes epidemics continued unabated. Further, these artificial chemicals may cause cravings: continually eating sweet foods, even if they have no calories, may lead us to crave other sweet foods that may contain sugar or starches.

Save dessert for special occasions. Most store-bought cakes, puddings, cookies, pies, mousses, ice creams, sorbets, candies, and candy bars are loaded with added sugars and should be eliminated from your diet. Even homemade versions made with added sugars should be an occasional indulgence, not a regular part of the meal. Birthdays, weddings, graduations, Christmas, Thanksgiving—these special occasions call for special treats. And most people celebrate with a birthday cake, not a birthday pork chop. The key word here is *occasional*. Dessert is not to be taken every day.

Choose seasonal fruits and dark chocolate. Many unprocessed whole foods contain natural sugars; for example, fruits contain fructose and milk contains lactose. A distinction is usually made between naturally occurring and added sugars because they differ considerably in amount and concentration. Fruits contain far less fructose than processed foods contain added sugar. Fruits also contain vitamins and nutrients along with a large amount of soluble and insoluble fiber (the pulp). This dietary fiber may act as an antidote to the harmful effects of fructose, and its bulking effect prevents overeating. So wherever possible, restrict your sugars to fresh seasonal fruits, preferably locally grown. A bowl of seasonal berries with whipped cream is a delicious way to end a meal. A small plate of nuts and cheese also produces a very satisfying end to a meal, without the burden of added sugars.

Dark chocolate with more than 85 percent cocoa, in moderation, is a surprisingly healthy treat. The chocolate is made from cocoa beans and does not naturally contain sugar, and dark and semisweet chocolate contain less added sugar than milk or white chocolate. Dark chocolate also contains significant amounts of fiber and antioxidants, such as polyphenols and flavanols. Studies on dark-chocolate consumption confirm they may help reduce blood pressure,[2] insulin resistance,[3] and heart disease.[4]

If you drink alcohol, choose low-carb wine or spirits. If drinking alcohol is part of your lifestyle, there are some options suitable for a low-carb diet. Choose wine with lower sugar content, typically dry white wines. Vodka is a low-carb spirit, but only if mixed with soda. Cocktails and other mixed drinks are not low-carb, and nor are beers and ciders. Like fatty acids, alcohol is metabolized by the liver, so if consuming alcohol, do so with meals and in moderation.

REDUCE REFINED CARBOHYDRATES

PLANT FOODS ARE richer in carbohydrates than animal products, but that doesn't mean you should avoid all plant foods. Unrefined complex carbohydrates, such as legumes (dried peas and beans), wild rice, vegetables, and unrefined fruits create a much lower insulin response in the body than refined carbohydrates, such as grain flours and the breads, cereals, and pasta made from them.

Eliminate refined grains and products made with them. When grains from the field are milled, the fiber is eliminated and the grains must be cooked to make them palatable. For example, whole-grain varieties of wheat such as farro, kamut, and spelt undergo less processing than grain flours, but any milling removes fiber (and often vitamins and minerals), which makes the refined grains significantly higher in net carbs than the original plants. Rice is another example. Husking and polishing the harvested grains removes (most) of their bran and husk layer to make them palatable for human consumption. However, these steps remove rice's natural fiber, and both white and, to a lesser degree, brown rice produce a significantly higher insulin response than the original unprocessed grain. Most cereals—corn, rye, sorghum, oats, barley, to name just a few—undergo similar processing before they reach the table.

Choose nonstarchy vegetables. Root vegetables, such as potatoes and sweet potatoes, are higher in carbohydrates than nonstarchy vegetables, such as spinach and cucumbers. However, root vegetables produce a lower insulin response than grains do because, unlike grains, they are normally consumed in their natural, unprocessed state. That said, choose nonstarchy vegetables more often than potatoes and other root vegetables, and eat them raw with as little preparation as possible.

Eat fiber-rich plants and seeds. When we talk about net carbs, we mean the total number of carbohydrates in a food minus the fiber. And the lower the net carbs, the lower the insulin response. Put another way, the more fiber in a carbohydrate-rich food, the lower the insulin response. Generally, dark leafy greens, such as kale and spinach, and nonstarchy vegetables, such as bell peppers and cauliflower, have the highest fiber and the lowest net carbs, and these are the vegetables to prioritize on an insulin-lowering (low-carb) diet. Spinach actually has a higher percentage of fiber than dried peas and beans!

There are two types of fiber, soluble and insoluble, and we need both. Soluble fiber dissolves in water and becomes a gel during digestion, which slows down this process (thus lowering the insulin spike after eating). Soluble fiber is found in the bran part of some cereals, nuts and seeds, legumes (dried beans and peas), and fruits and vegetables. It can also be taken in supplement form (e.g., psyllium husk). The fiber in chia seeds is largely soluble and makes a great replacement for grains, which is especially beneficial for people with metabolic syndrome trying to increase their fiber intake while decreasing their grain intake.

Insoluble fiber does not dissolve in water, so it adds bulk to the stool and helps food pass more quickly through the stomach and intestines during digestion. Insoluble fiber is found in the bran part of certain cereals and in some vegetables. Some foods, such as flaxseeds, can provide both forms of fiber. If milled, flaxseeds provide both insoluble and soluble fiber; whole flaxseeds only provide insoluble fiber. Insoluble fiber is a source of fuel (prebiotic) to nourish friendly gut bacteria (probiotic), which help to diminish pathogenic bacteria and build healthy gut flora.

MODERATE PROTEIN

PROTEIN GENERALLY PRODUCES a moderate insulin response—lower than carbs but higher than fat—but that response will be higher in people with insulin resistance. For example, type 2 diabetics and women with PCOS should eat enough protein to meet the daily requirements and avoid protein malnutrition, but no more than that.

Choose proteins carefully. There are both plant and animal sources of protein. Legumes are a good source of plant protein, but they are not necessarily recommended because they produce a higher insulin response than other good sources of plant-based protein, including almonds, chia seeds, broccoli, dark green leafy vegetables, and mushrooms. Recommended animal proteins include eggs, pork belly, chicken thighs, salmon, and sardines—all sources that produce a lower insulin response.

Some people include peanuts—actually a legume, not a nut—in a low-carb diet, but there are other concerns with peanuts, namely potential toxicity of nonorganic peanuts and "anti-nutrient" components. Soy products, such as tempeh, are also eaten by some people on low-carb diets. Like peanuts, soy also raises some concerns (possibly estrogenic effects, for one). I recommend choosing to consume the plant-based and animal proteins listed above.

Consume dairy products with caution. Certain animal proteins generate almost as much of an insulin response as carbohydrates, and the whey found in dairy (whether from cows, goats, or sheep) is one of them. Of all dairy products, milk has the highest amount of sugar (lactose). Milk is therefore generally avoided in a low-carb diet. And for better results, some people eliminate dairy products completely for varying periods of time. Avoid low-fat dairy products, which have a higher percentage of protein and/or carbs and thus will produce a higher insulin response than full-fat dairy. Instead, choose heavy cream (35 percent) and fermented dairy, such as yogurt and kefir, which are not only a good source of friendly gut bacteria but also lower in lactose. The "sugar" in these foods feeds the healthy bacteria, leaving the good stuff for us.

EAT MORE NATURAL FATS

FATS ARE DIVIDED into saturated, monounsaturated, and polyunsaturated fatty acids. We've long been told that saturated fats such as butter, rendered animal fats (e.g., lard), and coconut oil are high in calories and therefore bad for us. But books such as Nina Teicholz's *The Big Fat Surprise* and Gary Taubes's *Good Calories, Bad Calories* have revolutionized the way many people view fats. Of the three macronutrients (carbohydrates, proteins, fat), fat produces the least insulin response and thus is highly encouraged for a low-carb diet. Fat-rich foods contain the fat-soluble vitamins A, D, E, and K as well as water-soluble vitamins (e.g., B12) and minerals (potassium), all of which are needed for good health.

Avoid processed fats and trans fats. Refined fats such as margarine and vegetable and seed oils should be avoided. These polyunsaturated fats have been heavily processed and are highly inflammatory.

Choose natural full-fat foods more often. The conventional low-fat dogma has caused many people to be deficient in vitamins B12 and D, and many minerals, such as calcium, cannot be absorbed without fat-soluble vitamins such as vitamin D. Therefore, the best way to consume your broccoli (calcium) is with a healthy serving of olive oil (vitamin D). These fattier foods also contain the highest energy per gram and thus keep you feeling full longer. You might be surprised to learn that fat-rich foods normally have more nutrients than most grains, vegetables, or fruits. Foods such as eggs and beef liver are an almost complete multivitamin in and of themselves.

Table 12.1. Nutrients in animal foods versus in fruits and grains. RDA = recommended dietary allowance. Neg. = negligible. Bolding indicates the highest value among these foods. Data © Dr. Zoë Harcombe, www.zoeharcombe.com. Table adapted from the original with permission.

Nutrient (RDA)	Chicken liver	Sirloin	Eggs	Apple	Brown rice
	All values are given in RDA units, per 100 g of food				
Protein Quality	**149**	94	136	31	75
A (Retinol) (900 mcg)	**3290**	0	146	0	0
B1 (1.2 mg)	0.3	0.1	0.1	0	**0.4**
B2 (1.3 mg)	**1.8**	0.1	0.5	0	0.1
B3 (16 mg)	**9.7**	7.2	0.1	0.1	5.1
B5 (5 mg)	**6.2**	0.6	1.4	0.1	1.5
B6 (1.7 mg)	**0.9**	0.6	0.1	0.0	0.5
Folate (400 mcg)	**588**	13	47	3	20
B12 (2.4 mcg)	**16.6**	1.2	1.3	0	0
C (90 mg)	**17.9**	0	0	4.06	0
D (400 IU)	Neg.	0	**35**	0	0
E (15 mg)	0.7	0.3	1.0	0.2	**1.2**
K (120 mcg) (K1/2 not detailed)	0	1.2	0.3	**2.2**	1.9
Calcium (1000 mg)	8	27	**53**	6	23
Iron (18 mg)	**9.0**	1.5	1.8	0.1	1.5
Zinc (11 mg)	2.7	**3.9**	1.1	0.0	2.0

LOW-CARB DIET

THE LOW-CARBOHYDRATE DIET is what I recommend women with PCOS follow every day. For an occasional "detox," I have a stricter "fat and fiber feast" (see below). Most people associate a low-carb diet with eating bacon and eggs, which is a fair representation, but I like to characterize the diet as being high in fat and fiber rather than animal proteins. It is possible for the body to achieve ketosis from a plant-based diet. By definition, a low-carb diet means consuming foods that are low in carbohydrates (usually below 20 grams/day), moderate in protein (0.6 grams/kilogram of body mass), and high in natural fat (to satiety). Vegetarians who eat eggs, dairy, and nuts and pescatarians who eat fish and/or shellfish will have no trouble meeting these requirements. This diet is not about lowering calories; it is about lowering insulin. It is not about how much you eat, but what you eat and how often you eat it.

Principles of a low-carb diet

- Eat real food (avoid processed foods entirely).
- Eliminate added sugars and grains.
- Choose low-carbohydrate, high-fiber, nonstarchy vegetables.
- Eat natural, healthy fats and completely avoid refined polyunsaturated fats (eliminate margarine, vegetable oils, and seed oils).
- Aim for a diet that is 75 percent fat and fiber, 20 percent protein, and 5 percent unrefined carbohydrates.
- Eat full meals when hungry, until full (2–3 meals/day).
- Avoid snacks.

The low-carb diet is a rich and nutritious diet when followed properly. But it's important to seek proper medical supervision when you're on medication and/or changing your diet. The risks are associated with dehydration and/or hypoglycemia (low blood sugars), not malnutrition.

When switching to a low-carb diet, many people will go through a short induction phase, during which they may experience headaches, lethargy, nausea, confusion, brain fog, and irritability. This period usually lasts 2–5 days or up to a few weeks (until ketosis is reached) and is most often caused by dehydration and/or salt deficiency resulting from temporarily increased urination. Proper hydration (water and electrolytes) is recommended to mitigate these effects (see Beverages section below).

FAT AND FIBER FEAST

THE FEAST IS a temporary, more restrictive diet that's meant to be followed occasionally to reach a certain goal. For example, it's an easy way to transition to a low-carbohydrate and high–healthy fat diet with intermittent fasting because it is well defined and simple to follow. It often helps people to get over their cravings and other carb-withdrawal symptoms. The feast can also be a good way to prepare for longer fasts than you are used to by helping you reach a deeper fat-burning mode that will make the longer fasting periods feel easier. One of the most popular reasons to follow the fat and fiber feast is to "recover" from occasional indulgences during holidays or vacations.

Principles of a fat and fiber feast

· Emphasize the following fattier proteins: eggs (preferably free-range and organic); wild salmon and/or sardines; organic, pasture-raised bacon/pork belly; and fried or roasted animal skins/cracklings (pork, chicken, duck, turkey, etc.)
· Choose from the following fats and fibers: butter, ghee, olive oil, coconut oil, MCT oil,[5] avocado oil; rendered animal fats (lard, tallow, duck fat, etc.); avocados; olives; leafy greens (e.g., lettuce, spinach, bitter greens, kale, bok choi, etc.); fiber (chia seeds, flaxseeds, psyllium husk, konjac fiber).
· Always serve veggies with fat.
· Eliminate all dairy.
· Avoid all nuts.
· Season with spices and fresh herbs, to taste.
· Just like on the low-carb diet, eat when hungry and have full meals until you feel full.

What Should You Eat and How Much of It?

ENCOURAGED LIST

✔ Fat and fiber should be present at every meal and should compose the majority, about three-quarters, of the meal.
✔ Include as much natural dietary fat as you are comfortable with and to satiety.

Caution: Even though these are all-you-can-eat foods, only eat when hungry, stop when full, and do not overeat (this way you won't have to count calories). Keep these foods to full meals, and avoid snacking in between meals.

MODERATE LIST

≈ The remaining one-quarter of your meal is a moderate amount of animal protein, about the size and thickness of the palm of your hand at each meal. Eat full-fat dairy and nuts in moderation and always with meals.

Caution: Overeating protein is not recommended for people with insulin resistance. Dairy can often cause a higher insulin and inflammatory response in people who are highly insulin resistant, obese, diabetic, or have chronic inflammation and may have to be avoided by some for an indeterminate period of time.

Avoid all snacking, even on foods from the encouraged and moderate lists.

AVOID LIST

✘ This list contains all the foods to *avoid*, as they are either *inflammatory* foods (e.g., seed oils) or *carbohydrate-rich* foods (e.g., potatoes, rice, sugar) that produce a higher insulin response.
  I strongly suggest you avoid all the items on this list.

LEGEND:
✔ Least insulin response
≈ Moderate insulin response
✘ Highest insulin response

FATS

✔ Avocado
✔ Avocado oil
✔ Butter or ghee
✔ Coconut and MCT oil
✔ Macadamia oil
✔ Mayonnaise, full-fat and homemade
✔ Olive oil
✔ Olives
✔ Rendered animal fat (e.g., duck, lard, tallow)

HIGH-FIBER VEGETABLES

Most vegetables grown above ground

✔ Artichoke hearts
✔ Asparagus
✔ Bean sprouts
✔ Bell peppers
✔ Broccoli
✔ Brussels sprouts
✔ Cabbage
✔ Cauliflower
✔ Celery
✔ Chili peppers
✔ Cucumber
✔ Daikon
✔ Dill pickles
✔ Eggplant

- ✔ Green beans
- ✔ Kohlrabi
- ✔ Leafy green vegetables (e.g., spinach, Swiss chard, kale, lettuce, collard greens, rapini)
- ✔ Leeks
- ✔ Mushrooms
- ✔ Okra
- ✔ Pumpkin
- ✔ Radishes
- ✔ Spring onions
- ✔ Tomatoes
- ✔ Zucchini

PROTEIN

- ✔ Eggs
- ✔ Fattier cuts of meat (e.g., pork belly, chicken wings/thighs with skin, ribeye steak)
- ✔ Salmon and sardines
- ≈ Broths (e.g., bone broth)
- ≈ Game
- ≈ Lean cuts of meat (e.g., sirloin, filet mignon)
- ≈ Leaner fish and seafood (e.g., cod, sole, and shrimp)
- ≈ Offal (e.g., liver, heart, kidneys, tripe)
- ≈ Poultry

DAIRY

- ≈ Full-fat cheese
- ≈ Full-fat yogurt
- ≈ Heavy cream, 35 percent
- ≈ Kefir
- ≈ Sour cream
- ✘ Milk

NUTS AND SEEDS

Raw or as butters and milks

- ✔ Chia seeds
- ✔ Flaxseeds
- ✔ Brazil nuts, hazelnuts, macadamias, pecans, walnuts
- ≈ Almonds
- ≈ Pine nuts
- ≈ Pumpkin seeds
- ≈ Sesame seeds
- ≈ Sunflower seeds

✗ Cashew nuts ✗ Pistachios
✗ Chestnuts

FRUIT

≈ Berries (in moderate amounts)
✗ Apples
✗ Bananas
✗ Clementines
✗ Figs
✗ Grapes
✗ Guava
✗ Kiwis
✗ Lychees
✗ Mangoes
✗ Melons (e.g., cantaloupe, honeydew, watermelon)
✗ Nectarines
✗ Oranges
✗ Papaya
✗ Peaches
✗ Pears
✗ Pineapple
✗ Plums

SWEETENERS

Our clinical experience has demonstrated that people will have an insulin response to most if not all sweeteners, natural or otherwise (including stevia). People with more resistance to insulin (like type 2 diabetics and women with PCOS) will likely have an even higher insulin response.

✗ Agave
✗ Artificial sweeteners (e.g., acesulfame K, aspartame, saccharin, Splenda, sucralose)
✗ Candy
✗ Coconut palm sugar
✗ Erythritol (Swerve)
✗ Fructose
✗ Honey
✗ Malt
✗ Molasses
✗ Stevia
✗ Sugar (e.g., white, brown, cane, powdered sugars)
✗ Syrup (e.g., corn, high-fructose corn, malt, maple syrups)
✗ Xylitol

GRAINS

- ✗ All flours from grains (e.g., barley, corn, oat, pea, rice, rye, wheat flours)
- ✗ All forms of bread made from grains
- ✗ All whole grains (e.g., amaranth, barley, buckwheat, millet, oats, quinoa, rye, spelt, teff, wheat)
- ✗ Brans
- ✗ Breaded or battered foods
- ✗ Breakfast cereals, muesli, granola of any kind
- ✗ Cakes, biscuits, confectionary
- ✗ Corn products (e.g., corn chips, maize, polenta, popcorn)
- ✗ Couscous
- ✗ Crackers
- ✗ Pastas, noodles
- ✗ Rice and rice cakes
- ✗ Sorghum
- ✗ Thickening agents (e.g., gravy powder, cornstarch, tapioca, stock cubes)

ROOT AND STARCHY VEGETABLES

- ✗ Beets
- ✗ Butternut squash
- ✗ Carrots
- ✗ Legumes (e.g., beans, lentils, chickpeas)
- ✗ Onions
- ✗ Parsnips
- ✗ Peas
- ✗ Potatoes
- ✗ Sweet potatoes
- ✗ Turnips

BEVERAGES

- ✔ Black coffee
- ✔ Green tea
- ✔ Water
- ≈ Low-carb wine
- ✗ Beers, ciders
- ✗ Fruit juices
- ✗ Light, zero, or diet drinks of any description (contain sweeteners)
- ✗ Sodas
- ✗ Sweetened coffees or teas
- ✗ Vegetable juices

PROCESSED FATS

- ✗ Candy bars
- ✗ Commercial sauces, marinades, and salad dressings
- ✗ Hydrogenated or partially hydrogenated oils (e.g., margarine, vegetable oils, vegetable fats)
- ✗ Seed oils (e.g., canola, corn, cottonseed, grapeseed, safflower, sesame, sunflower oils)

PROCESSED FOODS

- ✗ All fast foods
- ✗ All processed foods
- ✗ Any foods with added sugar, such as dextrose, glucose, or high-fructose corn syrup
- ✗ Processed and luncheon meats

FAST INTERMITTENTLY

YOU'VE PROBABLY HEARD a lot about fasting lately, but in reality, people fast every single day and have been doing so since the beginning of time (whether they wanted to or not). Fasting simply means abstaining from food. As such, we all fast in between meals and when we're resting or sleeping, every day. And it is an ancient practice that has been used since the beginning of human time for survival, medical, religious, spiritual, and other purposes. Since all foods create an insulin response of some kind, fasting is the most accelerated and effective way to lower insulin levels (hyperinsulinemia) and restore insulin sensitivity (the opposite of insulin resistance).

Some people fast to achieve mental clarity. Others fast to improve their health and get off certain medications, such as drugs for the treatment of diabetes or hypertension. Others simply fast for weight loss and maintenance. A large part of the population still fasts for religious, cultural, or spiritual reasons. Women with PCOS may also benefit greatly from the various and flexible fasting schedules available. Because fasting lowers hyperinsulinemia more successfully and rapidly than any other dietary approach, this is a great tool to know and have.

Note that fasting is not recommended for women who are pregnant or breastfeeding. For those who are trying to conceive, fasting should be followed on a schedule based on the menstrual cycle and with proper supervision.

The relationship between fasting, insulin, and the low-carb diet

When the body is in a fasting or carb-restricted state, it burns fat. This natural physiological process is called ketosis. When the body burns fat (body fat or lipids from food), energy is released to all the cells in the body, including the brain. This means that we have the ability to produce energy even when we don't eat. Since it can normally take a few days to a few weeks to get into ketosis, it then follows that people who are already in ketosis (through a low-carb diet) would have a better time when fasting. Most people who eat a higher-carb diet in three meals a day, every day, have a ready supply of short-term energy stored as glucose (glycogen) in the liver. Therefore, it can take them several days or a few weeks of intermittent fasting to use up the short-term energy and get into ketosis. Remember, this supply of glycogen can be replenished during meals (depending on the amount of carbs and/or protein that are ingested). People already in ketosis (through a low-carb diet), however, can begin to burn fat almost immediately during their fasting periods, as they have no glycogen stores to burn up first.

Fasting means going into a nonfed state from a fed state. As such, we all fast during our normal day, in between meals and during rest periods. The most common periods range from just a few hours to longer periods such as 16, 24, 36, or 42 hours, and to periods of prolonged fasting such as two days or more. This idea may seem daunting at first, but after reading Dr. Jason Fung's blog on the Fasting Method site (www.thefastingmethod.com), watching his many YouTube videos, and reading his books, *The Obesity Code, The Complete Guide to Fasting,* and *The Diabetes Code,* you'll be well prepared!

Time-restricted eating, intermittent fasting, and alternate-day fasting

Time-restricted eating prolongs the period between meals. At its most basic, people stick to three large meals per day and abstain from food (fast) between meals (like we did back in 1977). Others extend their overnight fast to 16 to 18 hours and eat their two or three meals during a shorter "eating window" of six to eight hours. This type of fast is often referred to as intermittent fasting (IF). A 16/8 or 18/6 IF schedule means fasting for 16 or 18 hours, respectively, and eating during a period of 8 or 6 hours per day.

Alternate-day fasting (ADF) is used by many to accelerate their healing or progress by eating and fasting on alternate days. The most usual ADF schedules are 24, 36, or 42 hours. For example, on the 24h ADF schedule, people often eat two or three meals on their eating day, fast for 24 hours, and then eat one meal on their fasting day. They alternate between these eating and fasting days (see below) throughout the week. On a 36h ADF schedule, people often alternate between eating three meals on their eating day and eating no meals on their fasting day. On a 42h ADF, people alternate between eating two meals on their eating day and eating no meals on their fasting day. We refer to these meals as "breakfast," "lunch," and "dinner" for convenience, because it makes it easier for people to recognize the windows of time when they will be eating. Our clients mostly follow 16/8 IF, 24h ADF, or 42h ADF.

Table 12.2. Schedules for 16/8 intermittent fasting (IF) and 24h and 42h alternate-day fasting (ADF); X=no meal, M=meal, M/X=optional meal

16/8 IF	Mon	Tues	Wed	Thurs	Fri	Sat	Sun
Breakfast	X	X	X	X	X	X	X
Lunch	M	M	M	M	M	M	M
Dinner	M	M	M	M	M	M	M
24h ADF	**Mon**	**Tues**	**Wed**	**Thurs**	**Fri**	**Sat**	**Sun**
Breakfast	X	M/X	X	M/X	X	M/X	X
Lunch	X	M	X	M	X	M	X
Dinner	M	M	M	M	M	M	M
42h ADF	**Mon**	**Tues**	**Wed**	**Thurs**	**Fri**	**Sat**	**Sun**
Breakfast	X	M	X	M	X	M	X
Lunch	X	M	X	M	X	M	X
Dinner	X	X	X	X	X	X	X

Extended fasting

Abstaining from food for two days or more in a row is known as prolonged or extended fasting. People with severe metabolic syndrome, insulin resistance, and hyperinsulinemia—including obese women with PCOS—might benefit from longer fasting periods. However, extended fasting should always be practiced with caution and under proper supervision. Always consult your physician before making any long-term changes to your diet or eating habits.

Common concerns about fasting

Some of the most common concerns and fears around fasting are

·   slower metabolism,
·   dehydration, water, and/or electrolyte deficiency,
·   headaches and dizziness,
·   nausea,
·   cramps,
·   constipation or diarrhea, and/or
·   low blood sugars (hypoglycemia).

None of these conditions should occur if you are practicing fasting safely and with the proper knowledge and supervision. If you do experience any of these symptoms, particularly low blood sugar, consult a physician immediately. This is an emergency medical condition and must be addressed immediately.

Tips for fasting safely

·   Get informed (books, groups, medical professionals).
·   Stay hydrated (water and electrolytes, see below)!
·   Stay active.
·   Fit fasting into your lifestyle.
·   Play around with fasting schedules—exercise the fasting muscle!
·   Always stop a fast if you don't feel well.

Since intermittent fasting means abstaining from food for a period of time, liquids are not prohibited. In fact, I encourage you to always drink water. Green tea is also permitted, as it contains catechins that decrease hunger and increase energy expenditure.[6] Electrolytes such as salt and magnesium are highly encouraged, particularly if you are fasting for an extended period. Magnesium can be easily taken orally as a supplement (powder, liquid, or capsules) from your local drugstore at the recommended dose on the bottle. Salt is best taken in very small pinches under your tongue throughout the fasting day. I do not recommend salt in water as it can cause loose stools. Good sources of salt (like sea salts and celtic salts) are recommended. If you are on a sodium-restricted diet, consult with your doctor and make sure you are supervised throughout your fast. Although many programs advocate "fasting" with protein shakes and vegetable or fruit juices, I do not because protein, most fruits, and some vegetables create a moderate to high insulin response, which we are trying to avoid.

The liquids on the encouraged list (those with checkmarks on the following page) produce an insignificant or no insulin response and are highly recommended. The ones on the moderate list will produce a moderate insulin response and should be consumed one to three times a day, at most, if you are trying to extend a fasting period (we call these "fasting aids"). The avoid list includes beverages that will produce an undesired insulin response and should be eliminated from your diet completely during fasting periods.

What Fasting Aids Should You Drink and How Much?

ENCOURAGED LIST

✔ Water, flat or sparkling, whenever thirsty, average 8 cups/day
✔ Infused water, using lemon or lime, herbs (mint, basil), and/or fruit (do not eat the fruit)
✔ Apple cider vinegar, diluted in water
✔ Black coffee
✔ Green, black, oolong, and herbal teas
✔ Olive juice
✔ Pickle juice
✔ Pinch of salt (under the tongue or in water)

MODERATE LIST

≈ 1 cup bone broth (beef, pork, chicken, or fish; see page 183)
≈ 1–2 Tbsp chia seeds, soaked in water

≈ 1 Tbsp fat (e.g., olive oil, butter, MCT oil); try tea or coffee with 1 tablespoon of MCT oil, aka Bulletproof Coffee (see page 191).

≈ 1 tsp heavy cream
≈ 1 cup vegetable broth

AVOID LIST

✗ Artificially flavored drinks (e.g., Kool-Aid, Crystal Light, Tang; should not be added to water)
✗ Bouillon cubes (contain artificial flavors and monosodium glutamate or MSG—might trigger cravings and hunger)

✗ Fruit juices
✗ Naturally or artificially sweetened drinks
✗ Protein shakes
✗ Vegetable juices

MEAL PLANS AND SHOPPING LISTS
....

HERE I'M PROVIDING you with sample meal plans, shopping lists, and recipes for 16/8 IF (pages 144–147), 24h ADF (pages 148–151), and 42h ADF (pages 152–153) fasts. These are designed to get you started, but as you get more comfortable with the low-carb diet and as long as you follow the guidelines regarding what to eat and when to eat it, you can feel free to mix and match the recipes according to what you have in the fridge, what foods you like, or what you're in the mood to eat at any given meal. If you have food allergies or other restrictions, make sure to discuss them with your doctor.

Note that most of the recipes yield one serving. Why? We find that most of our clients are making these low-carb dishes for themselves rather than cooking for the whole family, and yet they can only find recipes that serve two to four people. In most cases, if you are cooking for more than one, you can simply increase the quantity of each ingredient and adjust the cooking times accordingly.

16/8 IF Schedule and Meal Plan

THIS INTERMITTENT FASTING schedule is also called time-restricted eating because it prescribes a 16-hour fasting period and an 8-hour eating window. This sort of schedule is usually followed most days of the week. Generally, we suggest two meals within that 8-hour gap.

If you are more ambitious, this can easily be modified to an 18/6 schedule, which is an 18-hour fast and a 6-hour eating window. For example, you might eat only between the hours of noon and 6 p.m.

There are other simple variations. If you find that you need to eat in the morning, then instead of skipping breakfast, you can eat breakfast and lunch and skip dinner. You may choose to eat within a 6-hour window with 8 a.m. breakfast and 2 p.m. lunch.

There is no "best" schedule. Choose the schedule that best suits your lifestyle. Many people eat dinner together as a family and will find that skipping dinner is difficult. However, from a physiological standpoint, it is best to eat most of your meals earlier in the day.

Sample Five-Day 16/8 IF Meal Plan; X=no meal

	Day 1	Day 2	Day 3	Day 4	Day 5
Breakfast	X	X ·	X	X	X
Lunch	Salmon Zpaghetti (page 170)	90-Second Sandwich (page 155) with Coleslaw (page 175)	Eggs Benny (page 164)	Guac Steak and Eggs (page 166)	My Tuscan Pizza (page 169)
Dinner	Egg Drop Soup (Home-made Bone Broth) (page 183)	Mexican Cauliflower Rice (page 168)	Stuffed Avocado (page 172)	Cabbage Spaghetti Bolognese (page 158)	Chicken and Avocado Salad (page 161)

SHOPPING LIST FOR 16/8 IF RECIPES

Meat, eggs, poultry, fish

- Bacon
- Boneless chicken thigh (with skin)
- Bones (e.g., beef, chicken, fish)
- Chicken feet
- Eggs
- Ground beef
- Steak (e.g., ribeye)
- Turkey breast slices
- Wild salmon (fresh)

Oils and fats

- Avocado oil
- Butter
- Extra-virgin olive oil
- Rendered (bacon) fat or lard

Produce

- Asparagus
- Avocados
- Basil, fresh
- Bell peppers
- Cabbage, white, green, and red
- Cauliflower
- Celery
- Cilantro, fresh
- Garlic
- Green onions
- Hot chili peppers
- Jalapeños
- Leafy greens (salad greens)
- Lemons
- Lime
- Onions, white/yellow and red
- Parsley, fresh
- Spinach, baby
- Tomatoes
- Zucchini

Canned/Nonperishable goods

- Black olives
- Sardines (canned in spring water)
- Tomato paste
- Wild salmon (canned, if not buying fresh)

Flours and baking goods

- Almond flour
- Baking powder
- Coconut flour
- Flaxseeds

Spices and condiments

- Apple cider vinegar
- Basil, dried
- Bay leaves
- Black pepper
- Cayenne pepper
- Cumin
- Garlic powder
- Garlic salt
- Mustard, prepared or powder
- Onion flakes, dried
- Oregano, dried
- Parsley, dried
- Red pepper flakes
- Rosemary, dried
- Sea salt
- Thyme, dried

Dairy

- Cheddar or Monterey Jack cheese
- Feta cheese
- Heavy cream, 35 percent
- Mozzarella
- Parmesan cheese
- Provolone cheese slices
- Sour cream

24h ADF Schedule and Meal Plan

THIS IS AN alternate-day 24-hour fasting schedule. A 24-hour fast generally runs from lunch to the next day's lunch, or dinner to dinner. Technically it may be slightly shorter than 24 hours but it is close enough. This sort of schedule is also known as a one meal a day (OMAD) way of eating. This may be done two to three days per week, but many people do well eating OMAD five or six days of the week.

In this example, you eat breakfast and lunch, then fast for 24 hours until the next day's lunch. Since this is the "fasting" day, you only eat a single meal. You would resume eating the next day at breakfast. Again, there are simple variations, and given most people's working day, a dinner-to-dinner fast is often most convenient. This means skipping breakfast and lunch on fasting days and only eating a single meal at dinnertime. This works well, because dinners are often eaten with friends and family whereas lunch and breakfast are less often social occasions.

Sample Five-Day 24h ADF Meal Plan; X=no meal

	Day 1	Day 2	Day 3	Day 4	Day 5
Breakfast	X	Cheesy Scrambled Eggs (page 160) with Berry Heaven (page 182)	X	French Toast Meal (page 165)	X
Lunch	Taco Soup or Salad (page 173)	Lettuce Wraps (page 167)	Cauli Fried Rice with Shrimp (page 159)	Butter Chicken (page 156)	Baba Ghanoush (page 181) with Seed Crackers (page 178)
Dinner	X	X	X	X	X

SHOPPING LIST FOR 24H ADF RECIPES

Meat, eggs, poultry, fish

- Bacon
- Bones (e.g., beef, chicken, fish)
- Chicken feet
- Chicken thigh fillets (with skin)
- Eggs
- Ground beef
- Meat or seafood (e.g., chicken thighs, steak, lamb, pork, shrimp, salmon)

Oils and fats

- Avocado oil
- Butter
- Cocoa butter
- Extra-virgin olive oil
- Rendered (bacon) fat or lard

Produce

- Avocado
- Bell pepper
- Cauliflower
- Celery
- Cilantro, fresh
- Edamame
- Eggplant
- Garlic
- Ginger, fresh
- Green onions
- Jalapeños
- Lemon
- Lettuce
- Lime
- Mixed berries
- Onion, white/yellow and red
- Parsley, fresh
- Red hot chilies, fresh
- Snap peas
- Tomatoes

Canned/Nonperishable goods
· Black olives

Flours and baking goods
· Almond flour
· Baking powder
· Chia seeds
· Coconut flour
· Flaxseeds
· Pecans
· Pumpkin seeds
· Pure cacao powder
· Sesame seeds
· Sunflower seeds
· Vanilla extract

Spices and condiments
· Apple cider vinegar
· Black pepper
· Cayenne pepper
· Chili flakes
· Chili powder
· Cumin powder
· Garlic powder
· Paprika
· Rosemary
· Sea salt
· Tahini (store-bought or make your own)
· Tamari sauce

Dairy
· Cheddar cheese
· Heavy cream, 35 percent
· Plain full-fat Greek-style yogurt
· Sour cream

42h ADF Schedule and Meal Plan

THIS 42-HOUR ALTERNATE-DAY fast allows two meals (lunch and dinner) on "eating" days and no meals on "fasting" days. Alternately, you could eat breakfast and lunch on eating days, and no meals on fasting days. The longer fasting periods allow more time for the body to metabolize its own fat.

Sample Five-Day 42h ADF Meal Plan; X=no meal

	Day 1	Day 2	Day 3	Day 4	Day 5
Breakfast	X	X	X	X	X
Lunch	X	Ribs with Bacon Bok Choi (page 174)	X	Chicken Fingers (page 162) with Bacon-Wrapped Fries (page 175)	X
Dinner	X	Spicy Sardines over Zucchini Noodles (page 171)	X	Avocado and Cream Cheese Cauli Sushi (page 155) with Salmon Wasabi Salad (page 177)	X

SHOPPING LIST FOR 42H ADF RECIPES

Meat, eggs, poultry, fish
- Bacon
- Chicken thighs (with skin)
- Eggs
- Ribs, beef, or pork

Oils and fats
- Avocado oil
- Butter
- Extra-virgin olive oil

Produce
- Avocado
- Cauliflower
- Cucumber
- Garlic
- Green onions
- Greens (e.g., bok choi, rapini)
- Parsley, fresh
- Shallots
- Tomatoes
- Zucchini

Canned/Nonperishable goods
- Nori paper
- Pickles
- Pork rinds
- Sardines (canned in spring water)
- Tomato paste
- Wild salmon (canned)

Flours and baking goods
- Almond flour
- Sesame seeds

Spices and condiments
- Apple cider vinegar
- Black pepper
- Chili flakes
- Cumin
- Dill
- Garlic powder
- Mustard, prepared or powder
- Onion powder
- Paprika
- Rosemary
- Sea salt
- Sriracha chili sauce
- Tamari sauce

Dairy
- Cream cheese
- Parmesan cheese
- Sour cream

Low-Carb Recipes

....

MAIN MEALS
....

90-Second Sandwiches
Avocado and Cream Cheese Cauli Sushi
Butter Chicken
Cabbage Spaghetti Bolognese
Cauli Fried Rice with Shrimp
Cheesy Scrambled Eggs
Chicken and Avocado Salad
Chicken Fingers
Egg Drop Soup
Eggs Benny
French Toast Meal
Guac Steak and Eggs
Lettuce Wraps
Mexican Cauliflower Rice
My Tuscan Pizza
Salmon Zpaghetti
Spicy Sardines over Zucchini Noodles
Stuffed Avocado
Taco Soup or Salad

90-Second Sandwiches

These sandwiches, made with bread modified from an old paleo recipe, are a new favorite for me. I dress the bread with butter, a slice of provolone cheese, and ham and serve it with a side of Coleslaw (page 175) or cherry tomatoes, olives, and lettuce leaves. *Serves 1 (two mini sandwiches)*

. . . .

> 1 egg, beaten
> 1 Tbsp almond flour
> ¼ tsp baking powder
> ¼ tsp salt
> 1 tsp ground flaxseeds
> 2 tsp butter
> 1 slice provolone cheese, cut in half
> 1 slice ham, cut in half

1. In a microwaveable mug, whisk egg, almond flour, baking powder, salt, and flaxseeds. Microwave on high for 90 seconds.
2. Invert and lightly tap the mug to release the bread onto a plate (caution: hot!). Cut bread into four slices, then toast (if desired).
3. Butter one side of each slice of toast. Top two of the buttered toasts with a slice of cheese and a slice of meat. Top with the remaining toasts to make two mini sandwiches. Serve immediately.

. . . .

Avocado and Cream Cheese Cauli Sushi

Cauliflower is versatile as a substitute for rice, and here it is in a Japanese recipe. If you own a sushi rolling mat, it will help you create tighter, more even sushi rolls. I pair this sushi with Salmon Wasabi Salad (page 177). *Serves 1*

....

2 Tbsp avocado oil

1 cup riced cauliflower (see Mexican Cauliflower Rice, page 168)

1 nori sheet (Japanese seaweed)

½ medium avocado, diced

1½ oz cream cheese, diced (about ¼ cup)

¼ English cucumber, diced

Sesame seeds, for garnish

Tamari sauce, for dipping

1. Heat avocado oil in a skillet over medium-high. Add riced cauliflower and cook for 5 minutes to soften. Remove from the heat and
allow to cool.
2. Place the nori on your sushi mat, if you have one, or on a piece of
plastic wrap.
3. Using damp hands, spread the cauli rice over the nori, leaving ¼ inch
free around the edges. Arrange avocado, cream cheese, and cucumber evenly across the quarter of the cauli rice nearest you.
4. Starting at the nearest edge, gently roll the nori around the filling,
using the sushi mat or your hands to tightly enclose the contents.
Dab a bit of water on the trailing edge of the nori to seal the roll.
Place the roll on a cutting surface, removing the sushi mat (if using).
5. Fill a tall glass with warm water. Carefully dip a very sharp knife in
the water, then pierce the nori and cut the roll into eight 1½-inch
sections.
6. Arrange the sushi on a platter and sprinkle with sesame seeds.
Serve with tamari sauce for dipping.

....

Butter Chicken

Mozambique, my country of origin, has three major culinary influences: Portugal, India, and Africa in general. I love all of them, and
butter chicken is one of my favorite Indian dishes. Pair this recipe with

Low-Carb Naan (page 176) or Turmeric Cauli Rice (page 179), and if you have additional butter chicken sauce, freeze it for later use with left-over chicken, meat, or paneer. *Serves 4*

....

Marinated chicken:

1 cup plain full-fat Greek-style yogurt

1 Tbsp lemon juice

1 Tbsp garam masala

2 tsp ground turmeric

1 tsp ground cumin

Salt, to taste

16 oz boneless chicken thighs, skin on

Cilantro, roughly chopped, for garnish

....

Butter sauce:

3–4 Tbsp butter or ghee (divided)

3 cloves garlic, minced

1 Tbsp grated ginger

Chili powder, to taste (optional)

2 medium tomatoes, diced, or 2 Tbsp tomato paste

Salt and pepper, to taste

1 cup chicken Bone Broth (page 183)

½ cup heavy cream (35 percent)

1. In a medium bowl, combine yogurt, lemon juice, garam masala, tur-meric, and cumin. Season to taste with salt. Add the chicken thighs, coating them completely. Cover and marinate overnight in fridge.
2. For the butter sauce, melt half the butter in a skillet over medium heat. Add the garlic and ginger (and chili powder, if using), and stir for about 1 minute to prevent the spices from burning.
3. Add the chicken and marinade and the tomatoes (or tomato paste) and season with salt and pepper. Pour in the bone broth and simmer for 30 to 35 minutes until the chicken is fully cooked.

4. Stir in the remaining butter and heavy cream and simmer for another 5 minutes.
5. Ladle the butter chicken into a bowl and garnish with cilantro. Serve hot.

. . . .

Cabbage Spaghetti Bolognese

This recipe is a low-carbohydrate adaptation of an old spaghetti recipe. Very filling and delicious! *Serves 2*

. . . .

2 Tbsp extra-virgin olive oil
¼ cup chopped onion
2 cloves garlic, minced
4 oz ground beef
2 eggs, beaten
Salt, to taste
1½ tsp Italian Spice Mix (page 187)
1 cup Bone Broth (page 183)
¼ cup tomato paste
2 cups shredded green cabbage
Chopped fresh basil, to taste
Drizzle of extra-virgin olive oil
Grated Parmesan cheese, for garnish

1. Heat a pan over medium-high and add the olive oil. Stir in the onions and garlic and cook for 2 minutes.
2. Add the ground beef, eggs, salt, and Italian spices and cook until the beef is browned, about 5 minutes.
3. Pour in the bone broth, stir in the tomato paste, and let the sauce simmer for about 7 minutes.
4. About 15 minutes before you plan to serve the sauce, bring a pot of salted water to a boil over high heat. Add the cabbage and cook until soft, about 7 minutes.

5. Heap the hot cabbage into a bowl. Ladle the sauce overtop, and serve hot with fresh basil, olive oil, and Parmesan cheese.

. . . .

Cauli Fried Rice with Shrimp

Cauliflower makes a great substitute for rice, and this Asian version with shrimp is delicious. Instead of using oil in my recipes, I often fry a couple of rashers of bacon and use its rendered fat to cook other ingredients. If you prefer, you can leave out the bacon and use 2 Tbsp of avocado oil or butter to stir-fry the vegetables. *Serves 1*

. . . .

2 Tbsp tamari sauce, divided
1 tsp grated fresh ginger
2 cloves garlic, minced
¼ tsp chili flakes
3 oz shrimp, peeled and deveined
2 rashers bacon, cut into ½-inch bits
   (or 2 Tbsp avocado oil or butter)
¼ cup chopped bell pepper
1 cup riced cauliflower (see Mexican Cauliflower Rice, page 168)
¼ cup edamame or snap peas
1 large egg, lightly beaten
¼ cup sliced green onions, for garnish
Sesame seeds, for garnish

1. In a medium bowl, combine 1 Tbsp tamari sauce, ginger, garlic, and chili flakes. Add shrimp, cover, and marinate in the fridge for a couple of hours or overnight, if you prefer.
2. Heat a large skillet over medium-high. Add the bacon (or oil) and heat, then stir in the shrimp, reserving the marinade, until well coated.
3. Add bell pepper, cauliflower, edamame (or snap peas), and marinade and stir-fry for 5 to 7 minutes or until shrimp are pink and firm to the touch.

4. Push the cooked ingredients to the side of the skillet and add the egg to the centre. Stir-fry until egg is well cooked, about 30 seconds.
5. Scoop the stir-fry into a bowl, setting the shrimp on top. Drizzle with the remaining tamari sauce and garnish with green onions and sesame seeds. Serve hot.

Cheesy Scrambled Eggs

I created this recipe as a mac 'n' cheese replacement for my kids. Instead of using cauliflower as a substitute for the pasta, I serve the cheese sauce over eggs, and I make it with butter, mascarpone, and Parmesan cheese for an "Alfredo" twist! *Serves 1*

Scramble:
2 rashers bacon, cut into ½-inch bits, or 2 Tbsp butter
3 eggs

Cheese sauce:
1 Tbsp butter
1 oz mascarpone cheese (about ⅛ cup)
1 oz grated Parmesan cheese (about 6 Tbsp)
Salt and pepper, to taste

1. For the scramble, line a plate with paper towels. Cook bacon, if using, in a skillet over medium-high heat until the fat renders. Transfer bacon to the plate to drain. Return the skillet to medium heat and add butter, if using instead of bacon.
2. Add eggs to the hot pan and scramble, stirring continuously for 30 seconds to a minute, until eggs are cooked but soft. Remove eggs from the heat.
3. For the cheese sauce, combine butter, mascarpone, and Parmesan cheese in a microwavable bowl and cook on high for 30 seconds. You can also cook these ingredients in a small pot over medium-low

heat until cheese has melted and sauce is creamy. Season to taste with salt and pepper.

4. Scoop the scrambled eggs into a bowl, pour the cheese sauce over-top, and gently fold the cheese sauce into the eggs. Sprinkle with bacon bits, if using, and shredded cheese. Serve hot.

Chicken and Avocado Salad

All low-carb salads are rich and filling. I keep prewashed leafy greens in my fridge so I'm ready to put a salad together in a couple of minutes. Any precooked meat or fish tastes great in a salad. I often add hard-boiled eggs, bacon bits, avocado, and a homemade dressing and voilà, salad. Here's a nice recipe. For a fancier presentation, layer the ingredients in the bowl instead of tossing them all together. *Serves 2*

Dressing (divided):
½ cup extra virgin olive oil
2 Tbsp fresh lime juice
¼ cup finely chopped fresh parsley
4 cloves garlic, minced
1 Tbsp finely chopped chili pepper
¾ tsp dried oregano
1 tsp coarse salt
Pepper, to taste (about ½ tsp)

Salad:
4 chicken thigh fillets, skin on
5 cups leafy greens, washed and dried
3 ripe tomatoes, sliced
½ red onion, diced or thinly sliced
2 avocados, pitted, peeled, and sliced
Fresh parsley leaves, for garnish

1. In a small jar, combine all of the dressing ingredients and shake until well combined.
2. Place the chicken thighs in a bowl, cover with half the dressing, cover, and allow to marinate overnight in the fridge.
3. Heat a barbecue or a grill pan to medium-high. Remove chicken thighs from the marinade and grill for 5–7 minutes on each side, until golden, crispy, and cooked through.
4. Remove from the heat and allow to cool slightly. Debone chicken, slice the meat into strips, and set aside. Reserve the bones for soup.
5. In a bowl, toss greens, tomatoes, onion, and avocado. Add the chicken and drizzle with the remaining dressing. Toss again and serve garnished with parsley leaves.

Chicken Fingers

The secret to delicious chicken fingers is to use juicy and succulent skin-on chicken thighs (and not chicken breast). The crunchiness is provided by a mix of Parmesan cheese, almond flour, and pork rinds, but any of these three on their own will work too. Pair this dish with a side of Bacon-Wrapped Fries (page 175) and Magic Dip (page 188). *Serves 1*

2 Tbsp extra-virgin olive oil, plus extra for baking
4 oz boneless chicken thighs, skin on
1 Tbsp almond flour
1 Tbsp ground pork rinds
1 Tbsp Parmesan cheese
¼ tsp salt
¼ tsp ground black pepper
¼ tsp paprika
¼ tsp ground cumin
¼ tsp dried rosemary

¼ tsp garlic powder
¼ tsp onion powder

1. Preheat the oven to 450°F. Drizzle a large baking sheet with olive oil.
2. Combine all the ingredients in a large resealable plastic bag and shake well to completely coat the chicken thighs.
3. Arrange the chicken thighs in a single layer on the tray and bake for 30 minutes. Turn chicken over and bake for another 15 minutes. Serve hot.

. . . .

Egg Drop Soup

Homemade Bone Broth (page 183) makes a great base for many soups, so I often make a batch and freeze it in one-cup portions so it's ready to use in all my soups and even gravies. Modify this Egg Drop Soup according to your tastes. For a bit of Asian flavor, add some tamari sauce. For a more Italian version, stir in some Italian Spice Mix (page 187) and tomato paste. It is easy to make and one of the most nutritious recipes around. Serve with buttered Seed Crackers (page 178). *Serves 1*

. . . .

1½ cups chicken Bone Broth (page 183)
2 tsp tomato paste (optional)
2 large eggs
Salt and pepper, to taste
1 Tbsp chopped fresh parsley or cilantro, for garnish
1 Tbsp chopped green onions, for garnish
Drizzle of extra-virgin olive oil

1. Heat the bone broth in a pot over medium-high and bring to a boil. Add tomato paste (if using). Stir to combine, then turn off the heat but leave the pot on the stove.

2. In a bowl, whisk the eggs. Slowly pour them into the steaming broth, whisking continuously. Season with salt and pepper, then stir the soup once more, cover the pot, and let sit for 30 seconds to a minute to cook the eggs.

3. Pour the soup into a bowl, garnish with fresh parsley or cilantro and green onions, and drizzle with extra-virgin olive oil. Serve hot.

Eggs Benny

Eggs Benedict is a classic dish of poached eggs over English muffins and drizzled with a delicious golden hollandaise sauce. Without the bread, this dish is pretty much low-carbohydrate, high–healthy fat. Luckily, 90-second bread (page 155) is a great substitute for English muffins. I've added some spinach to add nutrients and more fiber. Serve with cherry tomatoes and lettuce leaves. *Serves 1*

2 eggs
A few drops of white vinegar
90-second bread, sliced in half (90-Second Sandwiches, page 155)
1½ Tbsp butter, divided
½ cup baby spinach
2 cloves garlic, minced
Salt and pepper, to taste
2 slices ham or bacon
Hollandaise Sauce (page 185)
Sprigs of tarragon or other fresh herbs (optional)

1. Crack eggs into a bowl. Bring a pot half-filled with water to simmer over medium-low heat. Add a few drops of vinegar to the water, and using a fork or whisk, stir the water in a clockwise direction. Slide the eggs from the bowl into the pot and cook for 2 minutes, stirring gently without touching the eggs. Remove from heat and leave eggs in the pot for about 10 minutes.

2. While the eggs are cooking through, slice bread in half and toast.
3. Melt 1 tablespoon of the butter in a skillet over medium-high heat. Add spinach and garlic, season with salt and pepper, and cook until spinach has wilted.
4. Butter one side of each slice of toast and top with cooked spinach and a slice of ham or bacon.
5. Place a poached egg on each half and drizzle with Hollandaise Sauce. Garnish with herbs, if using. Serve immediately.

French Toast Meal

I don't always eat in the morning, but this traditional brunch recipe is a great way to "break your fast" at any time of day. It calls for using bread from the 90-Second Sandwiches recipe and bacon, but cook the French toast in melted butter instead of bacon fat if you prefer. Berries are a good fruit to have when trying to go low-carb, as they are lower in carbs and higher in fiber (and antioxidants) than other fruits.
Serves 1

2 rashers bacon, cut into ½-inch bits, or 2 Tbsp butter
1 egg
Pinch of cinnamon
Dash of vanilla extract
Splash of heavy cream
4 slices 90-second bread (90-Second Sandwiches, page 155)
⅓ cup heavy cream (35 percent), whipped, for topping
½ cup fresh berries, for topping
6–8 pecans, toasted, for topping

1. Line a plate with paper towels. In a skillet over medium-high heat, fry bacon, if using, until the fat renders. Using a slotted spoon, transfer the bacon bits to the plate to drain. Set aside the skillet with the bacon fat.

2. In a medium bowl, lightly beat egg, cinnamon, vanilla extract, and the splash of heavy cream.
3. Return the skillet to medium heat, and add butter if using in place of bacon. Dip bread slices in the egg mixture, coating both sides, and fry in the bacon fat (or butter) for 2 minutes. Turn the slices over and cook for another minute.
4. Transfer the cooked French toast to a plate, top with whipped cream, berries, pecans, and the reserved bacon bits.

. . . .

Guac Steak and Eggs

This dish is a staple for me. When eating out, I always ask for a fried egg on my steak. It's delicious. You can easily make this dish at home. Serve it with Pan-Fried Asparagus (page 177) and Hollandaise Sauce (page 185), raw cut veggies, or a salad (like Bacon Bok Choi, page 174). *Serves 1*

. . . .

4 oz rib-eye steak
2 Tbsp butter
1 egg
Guacamole (page 184)
Salt and pepper, to taste

1. Heat a barbecue or grill pan to high heat and grill your steak to perfection (rare, medium-rare, medium, or well-done, according to your preference). Remove from the heat, cover loosely with foil, and allow to rest for 5 minutes.
2. Melt butter in a skillet over medium-high heat. Reduce the heat to low, add egg, and cook for 1½ to 2 minutes, until white is cooked through. Cover with a lid and cook for 30 seconds more, or until yolk has set. Remove from the heat.
3. Place the steak on a plate and dress with Guacamole. Top with the fried egg and season to taste with salt and pepper. Serve hot.

Lettuce Wraps

Like the Stuffed Avocado (page 172), you can fill lettuce wraps with just about anything you have in the fridge (leftovers are great). Here I use a modified fajita recipe. I like leftover steak or ribs, but chicken thighs, lamb, pork, or shrimp all make great fillings. Use three to four ounces of your favorite. *Serves 1*

. . . .

2 Tbsp avocado oil
1 Tbsp lemon juice
¼ tsp ground cumin
¼ tsp garlic powder
¼ tsp chili flakes
¼ tsp paprika
Salt and pepper, to taste
3–4 oz meat or fish
½ bell pepper, diced
4–6 whole large lettuce leaves
1–2 green onions, chopped
Shredded cheddar cheese, for garnish
Guacamole (page 184), for garnish
Sour cream, for garnish

1. In a medium bowl, combine avocado oil, lemon juice, cumin, garlic powder, chili flakes, and paprika. Season with salt and pepper. Add the meat or fish, cover, and marinate overnight in the fridge.
2. Heat a large skillet to medium. Using a slotted spoon, add the meat or fish and the bell peppers. Discard the marinade. Stir and sear until the meat or fish is cooked through.
3. Arrange lettuce leaves on a clean, dry surface. Spoon one-quarter or one-sixth of the meat or fish filling onto each leaf. Garnish with green onions, cheese, guacamole, and sour cream, as desired.
4. Roll up each leaf to enclose the filling, or leave them open as "lettuce boats."

Mexican Cauliflower Rice

I love this recipe! Cauliflower is a great substitute for rice (and potatoes), and riced cauliflower is now available in many grocery stores. Alternatively, you can make your own riced cauliflower by finely chopping bits of cauliflower in a food processor. Store-bought seasonings such as Mexican chili powder often contain hidden sugars, so I always make my own. *Serves 1*

....

2 Tbsp avocado oil
2 cloves garlic, minced
3 oz ground beef
Salt and pepper, to taste
Red pepper flakes, to taste
½ tsp ground cumin
1½ cups riced cauliflower, fresh or frozen
¼ cup diced tomatoes
¼ avocado, sliced, for garnish
1 Tbsp minced jalapeño peppers, for garnish
1 Tbsp diced green onions, for garnish
10 black olives, pitted and diced, for garnish
1 lime wedge, for garnish
1–2 Tbsp shredded cheddar or Monterey Jack cheese,
   for garnish
2 Tbsp sour cream, for garnish
1 Tbsp chopped cilantro, for garnish

1. In a skillet, heat avocado oil over medium. Add garlic and ground beef and cook until meat is browned, about 5 minutes. Season with salt, pepper, red pepper flakes, and cumin.
2. When the meat is no longer pink, add cauliflower and tomatoes. Cook for 4 to 8 minutes (frozen cauliflower takes longer), then remove from heat.

3. Garnish the contents of the skillet with avocado, jalapeños, green onions, black olives, and lime wedge. Finish with the cheese, then cover the skillet and let cheese melt for 3 minutes.
4. Serve straight from the skillet with sour cream and cilantro.

. . . .

My Tuscan Pizza

There are thousands of low-carb pizza recipes made with almond flour, coconut flour, cauliflower, or even shredded chicken as a base. This one resembles a thick pancake. Pan-cooking the base saves time over baking it, and topping it with prosciutto, basil, goat cheese, and olives evokes the flavors of Tuscany. *Serves 1*

. . . .

Dough:
1 Tbsp almond flour
1 tsp coconut flour
¼ tsp baking powder
⅓ cup shredded mozzarella
Seasonings to taste (salt, pepper; Italian Spice Mix, page 187)
2 eggs
1 Tbsp organic butter

. . . .

Toppings:
2 Tbsp Pizza Sauce (page 189)
1 small tomato, sliced
2 Tbsp crumbled goat cheese
2 slices prosciutto
10 black olives, pitted and diced
1 handful fresh basil, roughly shredded
1 Tbsp extra-virgin olive oil and balsamic vinegar
Chili flakes (optional)

1. Place all the dough ingredients except the butter in a small bowl. Using a fork, mix until combined. (It will have the consistency of a pancake batter.)
2. Melt butter in a 6- to 8-inch skillet over medium heat. Pour dough into the skillet and allow to cook on one side for 3 minutes. Cover the skillet with a lid and invert the dough into the lid. Slide the dough back into the skillet and cook the second side for about 1 minute until fully cooked. Transfer the pizza base to a plate and let cool slightly.
3. If you prefer your toppings hot, preheat the oven to 350°F. Line a baking sheet with parchment paper and slide the pizza base onto it. Spread pizza sauce over the base, then arrange the tomato, goat cheese, prosciutto, and olives over the sauce. Bake for 10 minutes.
4. Serve the pizza topped with basil, drizzled with olive oil and balsamic vinegar, and sprinkled with salt, pepper, and chilies, if you like.

Salmon Zpaghetti

This recipe comes from my university days. At that time, I served it over spaghetti (obviously), but now I eat it with zucchini noodles, which I call zpaghetti or zoodles. It is a major comfort food, super quick to prepare, and just as delicious as I remember. *Serves 2*

2 Tbsp extra-virgin olive oil, plus extra for drizzling
¼ cup chopped green onions
¾ cup diced bell peppers
2 Tbsp tomato paste
1 large hot chili pepper, chopped (optional)
¼ tsp garlic salt
1 tin (7 oz) wild salmon in water, drained

Salt and pepper, to taste
¼ cup heavy cream (35 percent)
Zucchini Noodles (page 180)
1 Tbsp crumbled feta cheese, for garnish (optional)

1. In a skillet, heat the olive oil over medium; add green onions, bell peppers, tomato paste, chili pepper, and garlic salt; and cook for about 30 seconds. Stir in salmon and cook until warmed through. Season to taste with salt and pepper.
2. Just before you're ready to serve, stir in the cream for 2 minutes to warm and combine.
3. Mound zucchini noodles on two plates, ladle the sauce overtop, and finish with a drizzle of olive oil and/or feta (if using). Serve hot.

Spicy Sardines over Zucchini Noodles

This marvelous spicy sardine sauce is an old Portuguese favorite. Why sardines? These small, coldwater fatty fish are readily available and contain plenty of healthy omega-3 fatty acids. They're also a rich source of calcium, vitamin D, and other micronutrients. *Serves 1*

¼ cup olive oil (divided)
1 shallot, chopped
2 cloves garlic, minced
1 Tbsp tomato paste, thinned with a dash of water,
    or 1 medium tomato, diced
Chili flakes, to taste
Salt and pepper, to taste
1 tin (3¾ oz) sardines in spring water, drained
Zucchini Noodles (page 180)
¼ cup chopped fresh parsley and green onions, for garnish

1. Heat 2 Tbsp of the olive oil in a skillet over medium-high. Add shallots and garlic and stir-fry for about 30 seconds. Stir in the tomato paste (or tomato) and chili flakes. Season to taste with salt and pepper.
2. Stir in the sardines and the remaining olive oil. Season with more spice to taste.
3. Heap the zucchini noodles in a bowl, pour the sardine sauce overtop, and garnish with parsley and green onions. Serve immediately.

Stuffed Avocado

You can stuff avocados with pretty much anything (salad, meat, fish, seafood, eggs, bacon…) but my favorite filling is sardines and Homemade Mayo (page 186). *Serves 1*

1 avocado
1 tin (3¾ oz) sardines in spring water, drained
1 Tbsp Homemade Mayo (page 186)
1 hardboiled egg, peeled and roughly chopped
1 green onion, finely chopped
Salt and black pepper, to taste
Other herbs or spices (e.g., chopped fresh parsley, crushed chilies),
    for garnish (optional)

1. Cut avocado in half and remove and discard the pit.
2. In a small bowl, combine the sardines and Homemade Mayo. Add the egg.
3. Scoop half the avocado flesh into the sardine mixture and, with a fork, mash it in. Gently fold in the green onions. Season the mixture with salt and pepper.
4. Scoop the sardine salad mixture into the remaining avocado half. Garnish with herbs or spices, if desired. Serve immediately.

Taco Soup or Salad

This recipe provides two options! It can become a soup for cooler days or a salad for warmer ones. For the soup, you will need some home-made Bone Broth (page 183). For the salad, use lettuce instead. *Serves 1*

. . . .

3 oz ground beef

2 Tbsp extra-virgin olive oil, plus extra for drizzling

1 clove garlic, minced

1 tsp chili powder

1 tsp ground cumin

Salt and pepper, to taste

1½ cups beef Bone Broth (page 183) or 2 cups shredded lettuce

1 tomato, diced

Sliced avocado, for garnish

Sliced jalapeño peppers, for garnish

Grated cheddar cheese, for garnish

Sliced black olives, for garnish

Sliced green onions, for garnish

Sour cream, for garnish

Apple cider vinegar, to taste

1. Heat a skillet over medium heat, then add ground beef, olive oil, garlic, chili powder, cumin, and a dash of salt and pepper. Cook until beef is browned and remove from the heat.
2. For the soup, bring bone broth to a boil in a pot over medium-high heat. Add the beef mixture, stir in the tomatoes, and remove from heat. Ladle into a soup bowl and garnish as desired with avocado, jalapeños, cheese, olives, green onions, and sour cream.
3. For the salad, arrange lettuce in a salad bowl. Pour the beef mixture over the lettuce. Sprinkle tomatoes on top. Garnish with avocado, jalapeños, cheese, olives, green onions, and a dollop of sour cream. Drizzle with olive oil, add a splash of vinegar, and season to taste with salt and pepper, if desired.

SIDE DISHES
. . . .

Bacon Bok Choi
Bacon-Wrapped Fries
Coleslaw
Low-Carb Naan
Pan-Fried Asparagus
Salmon Wasabi Salad
Seed Crackers
Turmeric Cauli Rice
Zucchini Noodles

. . . .

Bacon Bok Choi

This side dish is tasty and hearty enough to be eaten on its own as a "main feature." But it makes a great accompaniment for eggs, tinned sardines, salmon, or steak. And you can use this recipe with bok choi or with other hardy greens such as broccoli rabe or rapini (my favorites), with bitter greens like mustard greens, or with spinach or kale. Save the delicate salad greens like lettuce for salads. If you prefer not to eat bacon or want a change, cook the garlic in 2 Tbsp melted butter or coconut oil and add a handful of nuts instead. I really like pecans or pine nuts with my greens. *Serves 1*

. . . .

2 rashers bacon, cut into ½-inch bits
2 cloves garlic, minced
1 bunch greens, thoroughly washed but left whole
Salt and pepper, to taste

1. Cook the bacon in a skillet over medium-high heat until the fat renders, about 5 minutes.
2. Add garlic and cook, stirring, for about 1 minute.

174

3. Add the greens, season with salt and pepper, and toss well to coat the greens in fat, bacon, and garlic. Cover with a lid and allow to cook for about 2 minutes.
4. Scoop the greens onto a plate, next to your protein and extra fat of choice.

. . . .

Bacon-Wrapped Fries

Whether you choose to wrap pickles or avocado wedges in bacon, these fries deliver a crunchy, salty punch that's delicious paired with a dipping sauce, such as Magic Dip (page 188), or with any crispy main dish, such as Chicken Fingers (page 162). *Serves 1*

4 pickles or wedges of avocado
4 rashers bacon

1. Preheat the oven to 425°F.
2. Tightly wrap each pickle or avocado wedge in a rasher of bacon. Arrange the "fries" seam-side down on a baking sheet and bake for about 10 minutes. Turn the fries over and bake for another 5 minutes on the other side. Transfer the fries to a plate and serve hot from the oven.

. . . .

Coleslaw

Unlike other salads, this popular deli side dish keeps well in the fridge for a few days, even once it's dressed. I often pack this coleslaw with leftovers from dinner for my lunch at the clinic the next day. *Serves 1*

1 cup mixed shredded white, green, and red cabbages
1 bell pepper, diced

1 stalk celery, chopped
1 green onion, chopped
2 Tbsp Homemade Mayo (page 186)

1. In a bowl, toss cabbage with bell pepper, celery, and green onions. Stir in mayo and mix gently until combined.
2. Cover and refrigerate until cold. Serve chilled.

Low-Carb Naan

This quick and easy flatbread recipe is an amazing way to enjoy Indian food and get your "bread" fix! Use naan to scoop up all the yummy sauce in your curry dishes, like Butter Chicken (page 156). *Makes 2 pieces*

1 Tbsp almond flour
1 tsp coconut flour
¼ tsp baking powder
Pinch of salt
Dash of Indian Spice Mix (page 187), plus extra for sprinkling
1 egg
Dash of heavy cream
3 Tbsp melted butter or ghee (divided), plus extra for brushing

1. In a medium bowl, whisk together the flours, baking powder, salt, spice mix, egg, cream, and 1 Tbsp of the butter to form a uniform batter.
2. Melt 1 Tbsp butter (or ghee) in a skillet over medium-high heat. Ladle half the batter into the skillet and cook for 3 minutes on one side, and then flip the flatbread and cook for another minute. Remove from the heat and set aside. Repeat with 1 Tbsp of butter (or ghee) and the other half of the batter.
3. Brush the top or both sides of the breads with butter and sprinkle with a pinch of Indian Spice Mix. Serve hot.

Pan-Fried Asparagus

Like the Bacon Bok Choi (page 174), this recipe is a staple for me. I was never a big fan of veggies, but now I love both stir-fried veggies and lots of salads. When paired with good fats (like butter, extra-virgin olive oil, Homemade Mayo, page 186, or Hollandaise Sauce, page 185), the good nutrients from the veggies are readily absorbed by the body. While fried asparagus is simple, adding Hollandaise Sauce makes it pretty delicious and fancy. Serve this asparagus as a side with any egg dish, including Guac Steak and Eggs (page 166). *Serves 1*

10–12 asparagus spears
3 Tbsp butter
Salt and pepper, to taste

1. Cut or break off and discard the woody stem end of the asparagus spears. Wash them thoroughly.
2. Melt the butter in a skillet over medium-high heat. Add the asparagus, season to taste with salt and pepper, and cook for about 5 minutes until the spears soften but retain some crunch and turn bright green. Serve hot.

Salmon Wasabi Salad

I particularly like this salad with Avocado and Cream Cheese Cauli Sushi (page 155). Adjust the heat to your liking by adding a bit of chili sauce. *Serves 1*

½ tin (3–4 oz) wild salmon, drained
¼ English cucumber, diced
½ avocado, diced
2 Tbsp Homemade Mayo (page 186)

1 tsp wasabi paste

1 tsp sriracha (optional)

1. Scoop salmon into a small bowl and add the cucumber and avocado. Toss to combine.
2. In a small cup, mix together mayo, wasabi paste, and sriracha, if using. Drop this dressing into the salmon salad and mix with a spoon until well combined.
3. Serve chilled.

Seed Crackers

I really like this low-carb cracker recipe because it is simple to make and it's a nice way to get some seeds into your diet. You can also vary the flavor by adding your favorite herb or spice; for example, ground paprika, cumin, or chili flakes or even chopped fresh or dried rosemary. I serve these crackers with butter or a low-carb dip, such as Guacamole (page 184), Baba Ghanoush (page 181), or Magic Dip (page 188). *Makes roughly 12–18*

3 Tbsp chia seeds

1 Tbsp sesame seeds

1 Tbsp pumpkin seeds

1 Tbsp sunflower seeds

1 Tbsp ground flaxseeds

1 Tbsp extra-virgin olive oil

1 Tbsp avocado oil

½ tsp salt

Freshly chopped or dried herbs or spices, to taste (optional)

⅓ cup water

1. Combine all of the ingredients in a bowl and let the mixture sit at room temperature for 15 minutes until the chia seeds create a pudding-like consistency.

2. Preheat the oven to 200°F and line a baking sheet with parchment paper (or have ready a silicone 12-hole muffin pan).

3. If you are using a baking sheet, place the pudding-like dough onto the baking sheet and cover it with a second layer of parchment. Using your hands or a rolling pin, flatten the dough until you have an even ¼-inch layer. Remove the top layer of parchment paper. If you are using a muffin pan, use a teaspoon to scoop a small amount of dough into the bottom of each muffin hole. Press it into a thin even layer.

4. Bake the crackers for 45–60 minutes until thoroughly dry but not burned. Remove from the oven and allow to cool. If the cooled cracker is soft and not crispy, return it to the oven at the same temperature for another 15 minutes or so and then allow it to cool.

5. If you baked the cracker on a baking sheet, break it into smaller, bite-sized pieces. If you baked the crackers in a muffin pan, invert the pan to release them.

6. Serve immediately or reserve in an airtight container at room temperature for up to two weeks.

Turmeric Cauli Rice

Cauliflower is the darling of low-carb cooking because it is very versatile. I steam it, roast it, and boil it, but I particularly like it riced. In this simple recipe, riced cauliflower is paired with an Indian spice (turmeric). Serve this quick and delicious rice with a low-carb curry, like Butter Chicken (page 156), to add some extra flavor. *Serves 1*

1 Tbsp olive oil, butter, or ghee
2 cloves garlic, minced
1½ cups riced cauliflower (see Mexican Cauliflower Rice, page 168)
1 tsp turmeric powder

Salt and pepper, to taste
Coriander seeds, for garnish (optional)

1. Heat olive oil (or butter or ghee) in a skillet over medium heat. Add the garlic and sauté for about 1 minute.
2. Stir in the riced cauliflower and turmeric and season to taste with salt and pepper. Cook for about 5 minutes until cauliflower is slightly softened.
3. Scoop into a bowl, garnish with coriander seeds, if using, and serve immediately.

....

Zucchini Noodles

Spaghetti is a side for many common dishes, so having this low-carb option is golden. Use these noodles to make Salmon Zpaghetti (page 170), Cabbage Spaghetti Bolognese (page 158), and Spicy Sardines over Zucchini Noodles (page 171). *Serves 1*

....

1 large zucchini
1 Tbsp organic extra-virgin olive oil, plus extra for drizzling
2 cloves garlic, minced
Salt and pepper, to taste

1. Using a spiralizer or a cheese grater, spiralize or grate the zucchini into long "zoodles." Set aside.
2. Heat olive oil in a skillet over medium heat, add garlic, and stir-fry for 30 seconds. Add zoodles and cook for another 30 seconds.
3. To serve, heap the zoodles in a bowl and ladle your favorite sauce overtop. Drizzle with olive oil and/or season to taste with salt and pepper.

PANTRY STAPLES, OR ABCDs:
APPETIZERS, BROTHS, CONDIMENTS, DRESSINGS, DIPS, AND DESSERTS

Baba Ghanoush
Berry Heaven
Bone Broth
Guacamole
Hollandaise Sauce
Homemade Mayo
Indian Spice Mix
Italian Spice Mix
Magic Dip
Pizza Sauce

Baba Ghanoush

This eggplant dish is most often known as a dip for veggies or Seed Crackers (page 178), but I often make it a main meal (and why not?). I just eat more dip, seeds, and veggies until I'm full. I prefer to roast the eggplant and garlic in the oven, but you can roast them over an open flame for a smokier flavor if you prefer. For a little heat, add a dash of cayenne pepper or paprika. *Serves 4 as a starter, or 1 as a meal (makes roughly 1 cup)*

1 medium eggplant
1–2 cloves garlic, unpeeled
¼ cup tahini (store-bought or make your own)
1 fresh lime, juiced, or more to taste
¼ tsp ground cumin
Salt and pepper, to taste
Cayenne pepper or paprika (optional)

2–4 Tbsp extra-virgin olive oil
Fresh parsley, for garnish

1. Preheat the oven to 450°F. Use a fork to pierce the eggplant all over so it doesn't explode while roasting. Wrap the eggplant and garlic separately in foil and place them on a baking sheet. Roast for 30 to 45 minutes.
2. Allow the roasted eggplant and garlic to cool slightly, then remove from the foil. Use a spoon to scoop out the eggplant pulp and some of the liquid into a bowl. Discard the skin. Use a knife to cut the top off the garlic cloves and squeeze the soft flesh into the bowl with the eggplant. Discard the skins. Allow the eggplant and garlic to cool to room temperature.
3. Add the tahini, lime juice, cumin, salt, pepper, cayenne or paprika (if using), and 1–2 Tbsp olive oil. Mash with a fork until well combined.
4. Season to taste with more salt, lime, cayenne or paprika, and/or olive oil.
5. Drizzle with olive oil and garnish with parsley before serving.
6. Will keep in an airtight container in the fridge for up to 4 days.

Berry Heaven

My low-carb desserts are always sugar- and sweetener-free. They normally consist of berries, whipped heavy cream, pure chocolate, and/ or nuts. Enjoy this treat after a meal. (If you prefer, pour the chocolate sauce into candy molds and allow to cool completely to make a "chocolate bar" or "coin.") *Serves 1*

1 oz organic cocoa butter
½ tsp pure (100%) cacao powder
¼ tsp vanilla extract
Pinch of sea salt

⅓ cup heavy cream (35 percent)

½ cup mixed berries

¼ cup pecans, roasted

1. Melt cocoa butter in the top of a double boiler set over medium-low heat. Add the cacao powder and remove from the heat.
2. Stir in the vanilla and salt and set aside.
3. While the chocolate sauce is cooling, whip the heavy cream until stiff peaks form.
4. Wash and cut berries and place them in a bowl. Drizzle with the chocolate sauce, then add a dollop of whipped cream. Garnish with pecans. Serve immediately.

Bone Broth

I use homemade bone broth for many recipes, including all my kids' soups, sauces, gravies, etc. Bone broth can be made in a slow cooker or on the stovetop—choose the method that best suits your lifestyle as the cooking varies depending on the type of bones used. Bone broth can be frozen in individual portions and kept for months, but if you run out or don't have time to make it, sourcing a very good store-bought one is also an option. Sip bone broth during your fasts too. *Makes about 12 cups*

2¼ lb raw bones (e.g., beef, chicken, fish)

2 Tbsp apple cider vinegar

½ lb chicken feet (optional)

1 onion, chopped

2 stalks celery

2 cloves garlic

1 bunch parsley

1 Tbsp sea salt

1 tsp black pepper

1. Preheat the oven to 450°F. Place the bones in a roasting pan and cook for 30 minutes.
2. Transfer the bones to a large pot, fill with cold filtered water, add the apple cider vinegar, and let sit for 30 minutes away from the heat.
3. Add the chicken feet, if using, and the onions and celery. Bring to a boil over high heat, then reduce the heat to a simmer.
4. Every 20 minutes for the first 2 hours, use a large spoon to skim and discard the impurities that rise to the top. Simmer another 10 hours for fish, 22 hours for chicken, and 46 hours for meat bones, adding more filtered water if needed so the pot is always three-quarters full. In the last 30 minutes before you remove the broth from the heat, add the garlic, parsley and spices.
5. Remove the broth from heat, let it cool, and then strain through a fine-mesh sieve. Discard the solids.
6. Divide the broth into 1-cup containers and freeze. (If you prefer, allow the broth to cool, skim and discard the fat from the top, and then freeze the broth.)
7. To use, reheat the broth in a slow cooker or on the stove on medium-high. Sip or use in recipes that call for stock or broth.

Guacamole

Everybody loves guacamole. It can be used as a spread on just about any food and can be served as a dip, salad dressing, or garnish for a meat or fish dish. *Serves 2*

1 ripe avocado
2 Tbsp chopped green onions
½ tsp lemon or lime juice or apple cider vinegar
¼ ripe tomato, chopped (can remove seeds and pulp)
¼ red onion, chopped
2 Tbsp extra-virgin olive oil

½ tsp salt
Dash of black pepper
1 chili, seeded and minced
2 Tbsp chopped cilantro

1. Cut the ripe avocado in half and remove and discard the pit. With a large spoon, scoop the avocado flesh into a bowl. Mash with a fork until smooth.
2. Add the remaining ingredients and blend well.
3. Serve chilled or at room temperature. Will keep in the fridge, covered with plastic wrap pressed tight to the surface (so it doesn't oxidize), for a couple of days.

Hollandaise Sauce

This delicious and nutritious golden sauce is traditionally served over poached eggs (Eggs Benny, page 164), vegetables (e.g., asparagus), or steak. This recipe is made using a double boiler, but you can try using a microwave as an easier and quicker option. *Serves 1*

1 egg yolk
½ tsp lemon juice
2 Tbsp butter, melted
Pinch of salt
Cayenne or black pepper, to taste

1. In a stainless steel bowl, vigorously whisk the egg yolk and lemon juice together until the mixture thickens and doubles in volume.
2. Place the egg mixture in the top of a double boiler set over medium-low heat. Slowly drizzle the melted butter into the egg mixture, while whisking continuously. Continue whisking until the sauce thickens and doubles in volume.

3. Remove from the heat and whisk in salt and pepper.
4. Serve hot. If the sauce gets too thick as it cools, whisk in a few drops of warm water before serving.

Homemade Mayo

I keep this mayo on hand all the time because it's quick and easy to make with a hand blender (a whisk and a bowl will work fine if you don't have a hand blender). This version is not as strongly flavored as traditional mayonnaise recipes that are made with olive oil, which means I can easily use it as a dip, salad dressing, or base for other dressings (e.g., Salmon Wasabi Salad, page 177). Often I make mayo on Monday and it lasts in the fridge till Friday. *Makes a little over 1 cup, about 8 servings*

1 whole egg
1 tsp lemon juice or apple cider vinegar
¼ tsp mustard, prepared or powder
Pinch of salt and black pepper
1 cup avocado oil

1. Place the egg, lemon juice, mustard, salt, and pepper in the bottom of a hand-blender cup, hold the blender flush with the bottom of the cup, and mix for 30 seconds.
2. With the blender going, slowly drizzle in the oil, always keeping the blender flush with the bottom of the cup. Once mayo emulsifies (about 2 minutes), stop mixing, remove the blender, unplug it, and use a spatula to scrape any mayo left on the blender into the cup.
3. If you do not have a hand blender, whisk together all the ingredients except the oil in a medium bowl.
4. Slowly drizzle in the oil while whisking constantly. If oil is added too quickly, the mixture will not emulsify.
5. Will keep in an airtight container in the fridge for up to 5 days.

Indian Spice Mix

I like to make spice mixes myself rather than buying store-bought ones, and this one is useful because I make a lot of Indian-style dishes. It's a great base for a curry, or even to sprinkle on naan. Add some heat to the mix by using the chili flakes, or leave them out. It's up to you! To simplify this recipe, combine equal parts store-bought curry powder, garam masala, cumin, coriander, and salt. *Makes ⅛ cup*

1 tsp ground cumin
1 tsp ground coriander
½ tsp ground turmeric
½ tsp ground ginger
½ tsp sea salt
Pinch of ground cinnamon
Pinch of ground cardamom
Pinch of ground cloves
Chili flakes, to taste

Mix all the ingredients in a small bowl until well combined. Transfer to an airtight container, like a glass jar or a resealable bag, and store at room temperature for up to 3 months.

Italian Spice Mix

Most prepared spice mixes and even many do-it-yourself recipes call for added sugar. There is no need, as the spices provide plenty of flavor. Prepare the spice mix ahead of time and use it whenever more flavor is needed. *Makes ⅓ cup*

1 tsp salt
1 Tbsp dried parsley

¼ tsp dried thyme

2 tsp dried onion flakes

2 tsp garlic powder

1 tsp finely crushed bay leaf

1 Tbsp dried oregano

1 Tbsp dried basil

2 tsp dried rosemary

Mix all the ingredients in a small bowl until well combined. Transfer to an airtight container, like a glass jar or a resealable bag, and store at room temperature for up to 3 months.

Magic Dip

I call this my Magic Dip because as long as I serve this with her meals, my "picky eater" will eat almost anything. Magic! It is especially good with veggies, cracklings, or Bacon-Wrapped Fries (page 175). *Serves 1*

¼ cup sour cream

½ tsp dried dill

¼ tsp garlic powder

¼ tsp onion powder

Salt and pepper, to taste

1. Mix all the ingredients in a small bowl until well combined.
2. Will keep in an airtight container in the fridge for up to 4 days.

Pizza Sauce

Like other store-bought condiments, pizza sauce tends to be made with added sugar. This recipe uses tomato paste to make a very quick sauce, but if you have more time, search out a more elaborate family recipe made without sugar or refined carbohydrates. You can multiply this recipe, depending on the number of servings you're making. *Serves 1*

1 Tbsp extra-virgin olive oil
2 Tbsp tomato paste
½ tsp Italian Spice Mix (page 187)

1. Heat the olive oil in a skillet over medium heat and add the tomato paste and spice mix. Simmer the sauce for about 3 minutes. Allow to cool before using or storing.
2. Will keep in an airtight container in the fridge for 4 days or in the freezer for several months. Thaw before use.

BEVERAGES

. . . .

These drinks can be enjoyed during meals or fasting periods. Drinks that contain nutrients like nut milks (e.g., Iced Coconut Matcha Latte) should be paired with meals; all other drinks (e.g., Ginger Green Detox Tea) can be enjoyed liberally between meals and during fasting periods.

ACV Mix
Alcohol-Free Margarita
Bulletproof Coffee
Flavored Sparkling Water
Green Tea Recipes
    Decaf Ginger Citrus Latte (Digestion Elixir)
    Decaf Vanilla Rooibos Latte (Immunity Elixir)
    Earl Grey Latte
    Ginger Green Detox Tea
    Iced Coconut Matcha Latte
    Matcha Fasting Aid
Infused Water
Virgin "Dirty" Martini

ACV Mix

If made properly, this apple cider vinegar (ACV) drink should taste just like pickle juice. Use any natural salt; coarse salt refers to Himalayan pink salt, sea salt, kosher salt, or Maldon salt. You can also add fresh dill (or dried, if that's all you have) for taste. *Serves 1*

    1–2 Tbsp apple cider vinegar
    1 cup water
    1 tsp coarse salt

Fresh or dried dill, to taste (optional)

Ice, to taste

Stir together the vinegar, water, and salt until the salt dissolves. Season with dill, if using. Add the ice and pour into a drinking glass.

. . . .

Alcohol-Free Margarita

During fasting periods, taking a pinch of salt every once in a while helps prevent dehydration and headaches. Drinking a "margarita" is a good way to take your salt! Note that this drink is tart, not sweet. *Serves 1*

½ cup ice

¼ cup freshly squeezed lemon juice

¼ cup unflavored sparkling water

¼ tsp coarse salt

Lime wedge

1. Rim a margarita glass with salt and place it in the freezer to chill for a couple of hours.
2. In a blender, combine ice, lemon juice, sparkling water, and salt until ice is crushed.
3. Pour into the salt-rimmed glass and serve with a wedge of lime.

. . . .

Bulletproof Coffee

There are many recipes for this drink, also known as keto coffee. It combines high-quality coffee beans, butter, and medium-chain triglycerides (MCT) derived from 100 percent pure coconut oil. For a decaf version, use decaf coffee or decaffeinated herbal teas. *Serves 1*

1 Tbsp MCT oil
1 Tbsp unsalted butter, room temperature
1 cup coffee, hot

1. Place all the ingredients in a blender and process until creamy. The drink should look like a cappuccino.
2. Pour into a mug and serve hot (cold coffee will separate).

Flavored Sparkling Water

Make your own flavored carbonated water without sweeteners. I like this version with lemon and mint, which reminds me of a "virgin" mojito. But use any tart citrus fruits, berries, or vegetables you like, including lime, strawberries, or cucumber. Do not eat them if you are fasting.

If you have a SodaStream machine, you can make your own sparkling water at home. (And if you don't like fizzy drinks, see Infused Water, page 197.) *Serves 1*

1 cup unflavored sparkling water
1 Tbsp freshly squeezed lemon juice
2 lemon wedges
2–3 mint leaves
Ice, to taste

1. Pour the sparkling water into a drinking glass and stir in the lemon juice, lemon wedges, mint leaves, and ice.
2. Serve immediately, or allow it to infuse for a few minutes to enhance the flavor.

Decaf Ginger Citrus Latte (Digestion Elixir)

Used in traditional Chinese medicine for its digestive and anti-inflammatory properties, ginger—when combined with citrus peel and licorice root—is especially helpful for suppressing appetite and controlling grazing and cravings. *Serves 1*

....

1 cup water
1 sachet Ginger Citrus–flavored green tea crystals
½ tsp ghee or coconut butter
¼ cup macadamia (or other) nut milk
Himalayan pink salt (optional)

1. Heat the water in a small pot over medium-low. Do not allow it to boil.
2. Place the tea crystals in a small bowl, add the hot water, and stir well. Pour the tea mixture into a glass.
3. In a separate glass, combine ghee (or coconut butter) with nut milk and froth with a hand-held frother or blender until smooth.
4. Pour over the tea, mix well, and serve immediately.

Decaf Vanilla Rooibos Latte (Immunity Elixir)

Rooibos is a red herbal tea native to South Africa, and because it is especially high in two antioxidants that promote gut health and boost immunity, I call this an Immunity Elixir. *Serves 1*

....

1 cup water
1 sachet Vanilla Rooibos–flavored green tea crystals
½ tsp ghee or coconut butter
¼ cup macadamia (or other) nut milk

1. Heat the water in a small pot over medium-low. Do not allow it to boil.
2. Place the tea crystals in a small bowl, add the hot water, and stir well. Pour the tea mixture into a glass.
3. In a separate glass, combine ghee (or coconut butter) with nut milk and froth with a hand-held frother or hand blender until smooth.
4. Pour over the tea, mix well, and serve immediately.

. . . .

Earl Grey Latte

Looking for a bulletproof tea instead of coffee? Here's a wonderful option with the delicious flavors of cocoa and vanilla. *Serves 1*

. . . .

1 cup water
1 sachet Earl Grey green tea crystals
½ tsp vanilla extract
½ tsp cacao powder
½ tsp ghee, coconut butter, or coconut oil
¼ cup macadamia (or other) nut milk

1. Heat the water in a small pot over medium-low. Do not allow it to boil.
2. Place the tea crystals in a small bowl, add the hot water, and stir well. Add vanilla extract and cacao powder and stir again. Pour the tea mixture into a glass.
3. In a separate glass, combine ghee (or coconut butter or oil) with nut milk and froth with a hand-held frother or a hand blender until smooth.
4. Pour over the tea, mix well, and serve immediately.

Ginger Green Detox Tea

In traditional Chinese medicine, ginger has "warming properties" and is good for digestion. As such, this beverage pairs well with any meal above. Green tea catechins are touted for their weight-loss properties as well as in aiding appetite suppression, making green tea a great fasting aid. *Serves 1*

¼ cup water
1 sachet Ginger Green Fasting Tea crystals
2 Tbsp apple cider vinegar
Dash of Himalayan pink salt
½ cup ice cubes
Mint leaves, for garnish

1. Heat the water in a small pot over medium-low. Do not allow it to boil. Place the tea crystals in a glass, add the hot water, apple cider vinegar, and pink salt, and stir to combine.
2. Add the ice and stir gently to combine. Garnish with mint leaves and serve.

Iced Coconut Matcha Latte

Matcha green tea has long been used as a health aid due to its antioxidant properties, but it can also be a great "fasting aid" for its hunger-suppressing power. This beverage can be enjoyed with a meal (such as Eggs Benny, page 164) or on a fasting day. *Serves 1*

½ cup water
1 sachet Matcha Green Fasting Tea crystals
1 tsp ghee
2 tsp MCT oil

1 cup crushed ice
½ cup coconut milk
¼ tsp pure vanilla extract

1. Heat the water in a small pot over medium-low. Do not allow it to boil.
2. Place the tea crystals in a small bowl, add 1 Tbsp of the hot water, and stir to form a paste.
3. Pour the remaining hot water, ghee, and MCT oil into the matcha paste and blend with a hand blender or a whisk. Add more hot water if you prefer a thinner consistency. Pour the tea mixture into a glass.
4. Add the crushed ice and stir gently to combine.
5. In a separate glass, use a hand-held frother or a hand blender to combine the coconut milk and vanilla. Pour over the iced tea mixture and serve immediately.

Matcha Fasting Aid

Matcha is a powdered green tea that can be whisked into hot water to form a frothy drink. Originally from China and Japan, matcha contains the most catechins of any tea. Catechins are excellent for helping to suppress cravings, provide satiety, and boost energy. *Serves 1*

1 sachet Matcha Green Fasting Tea crystals
2 cups water
Ice
Squeeze of lemon or orange juice

1. Heat the water in a small pot over medium-low. Do not allow it to boil.
2. Place the tea crystals in a small bowl, add the hot water, and froth or stir until fully blended.
3. Add ice and a squeeze of lemon or orange. Mix well and serve.

Infused Water

Infused waters are so popular that special containers can be purchased for the purpose of making them. But you can easily infuse fruits, vegetables, and garden herbs in a regular drinking glass, carafe, or other container. (Do not eat the fruits or vegetables during fasting periods.) *Serves 1*

. . . .

1 cup water
¼ cup fresh or frozen berries (your favorite, or a mix)
½ English cucumber, sliced
Fresh basil leaves
Ice, to taste

1. Pour the water into an infuser or a drinking glass and stir in the berries, cucumber, basil leaves, and ice.
2. Allow the water to infuse in the fridge (if you like cold water) or at room temperature (if you are like me) for an hour before serving.

Virgin "Dirty" Martini

I discovered this drink on a fasting day. Lots of people drink pickle juice during their fasts, but I personally prefer the taste of olives. Use the brine from any type of bottled olives in this recipe; you can also buy prepackaged olive brine (sometimes called olive juice), or make your own. Strain the olives from the brine before using. *Serves 1*

. . . .

½ cup ice
½ cup olive brine
Olives, for garnish

1. Place a martini glass in the freezer to chill for a couple of hours.
2. If you own a cocktail shaker, throw in the ice and pour the olive

brine over it. Close the mixer and shake vigorously for about 10 seconds. Pour into the martini glass.

3. If you don't have a shaker, pour the brine into the martini glass and add the ice. Stir.

4. Garnish with olives before serving.

JESSICA

Jessica accompanied her mom to her first appointment with me and decided right there and then that she wanted to become my patient too. She had a BMI in the overweight range and wanted to lose weight. Right away she began to follow a strict low-carb diet with intermittent fasting, alternating three 24-hour fasts per week with 16-hour fasts. Essentially, Jessica ate two meals one day and one meal the next day, alternating like this for a month. At the end of the 30 days, Jessica had lost 4 inches (10 centimeters) from around her waist and 7.7 pounds (3.5 kilograms) overall. She was thrilled and so was I. Though I didn't know it at the time, Jessica was a newlywed trying to conceive despite a history of irregular periods.

Just four months later—and after the Christmas holidays, no less—Jessica had completed a five-day fast, had lost a total of 11 pounds (5 kilograms), and had a BMI at the high end of the normal range. On her very next menstrual cycle, Jessica got pregnant! Once she'd nearly reached her first trimester, Jessica let me know she was pregnant and we spoke about what kind of program she should follow during the remainder of her pregnancy. Jessica's mom had had gestational diabetes during her pregnancy, and Jessica was concerned that she too might be at risk. I advised her to stop fasting, but to continue on a low-carb diet, eating when hungry and continuing until full. I also advised her to avoid snacking.

I saw Jessica again when she was 19 weeks pregnant. She'd stopped following a low-carb diet, was snacking, and had gained 13.2 pounds (6 kilograms). She was concerned about such a large weight gain in so short a period, and so was I. Again I advised her not to fast, but to continue on a low-carb diet, eating when hungry and continuing until full. Just seven weeks later, as both of us had feared, Jessica was diagnosed with gestational diabetes.

She'd gained a total of 24.6 pounds (11.2 kilograms) in less than six months of pregnancy, or nearly double what doctors suggest is healthy. Jessica's doctor told her she would likely need medication to control her diabetes. It was a wakeup call.

Within a week of restarting a low-carb diet (with proper electrolytes), Jessica's fasting blood glucose returned to normal, which suggests she had reversed her gestational diabetes, and she had more energy, felt better, slept better, and had many fewer sugar cravings. Jessica had no further complications throughout her pregnancy and delivered a healthy baby boy.

Jessica successfully lost her baby weight, and once she stopped breastfeeding, she slowly transitioned from eating three full meals per day back to her regular combination of 24-hour alternate-day fasting and 16-hour intermittent fasting.

Metric
Conversion Chart

....

Volume	
Imperial	**Metric**
¼ tsp	1 mL
½ tsp	2.5 mL
¾ tsp	4 mL
1 tsp	5 mL
1½ tsp	7.5 mL
1 Tbsp	15 mL
1½ Tbsp	22 mL
2 Tbsp	30 mL
3 Tbsp	45 mL
¼ cup	60 mL
⅓ cup	80 mL
½ cup	125 mL
⅔ cup	160 mL
¾ cup	185 mL
1 cup	250 mL

Weight	
Imperial	**Metric**
½ oz	15 g
1 oz	30 g

Weight	
Imperial	Metric
1½ oz	45 g
2 oz	60 g
3 oz	85 g
4 oz / ¼ lb	115 g
8 oz / ½ lb	225 g
12 oz / ¾ lb	340 g
16 oz / 1 lb	450 g

Length	
Imperial	Metric
¼ inch	6 mm
½ inch	1.2 cm
1 inch	2.5 cm
1½ inches	4 cm
2 inches	5 cm
4 inches	10 cm
6 inches	15 cm
8 inches	20 cm

Oven Temperature	
Imperial	Metric
200°F	95°C
325°F	160°C
350°F	180°C
400°F	200°C
425°F	220°C
450°F	230°C

Tin Sizes	
Imperial	Metric
3¾ oz	125 g
7 oz	198 g

Notes

....

Introduction: The Many Faces of Polycystic Ovary Syndrome

1 Sirmans SM, Pate KA. Epidemiology, diagnosis, and management of polycystic ovary syndrome. Clin Epidemiol. 2014; 6: 1–13.

Chapter 1: The Diabetes of Bearded Women

1 This quote and the ones in the next paragraph from: Azziz R et al. Polycystic ovary syndrome: an ancient disorder? Fertil Steril. 2011 Apr; 95(5): 1544–8.

2 Insler V, Lunesfeld B. Polycystic ovarian disease: a challenge and controversy. Gynecol Endocrinol. 1990; 4: 51–69.

3 Brown, WH. A case of pluriglandular syndrome: "diabetes of bearded women." Lancet. 1928 Nov; 212(5490): 1022–3.

4 Stein IF, Leventhal ML. Amenorrhoea associated with bilateral polycystic ovaries. Am J Obstet Gynecol. 1935; 29: 181–91.

5 Redrawn from a figure in Kovacs GT, Norman R, eds. Polycystic ovary syndrome, 2nd ed. New York: Cambridge University Press; 2007.

6 Stein IF et al. Results of bilateral ovarian wedge resection in 47 cases of sterility. Am J Obstet Gynecol. 1949; 58(2): 267–73.

7 Swanson M et al. Medical implications of ultrasonically detected polycystic ovaries. J Clin Ultrasound. 1981; 9: 219–22.

8 Redrawn from a figure in Diamanti-Kandarakis E, Dunaif A. Insulin resistance and the polycystic ovary syndrome revisited: an update on mechanisms and implications. Endocr Rev. 2012 Dec; 33(6): 981–1030.

9 Ibid.

10 Sirmans SM, Pate KA. Epidemiology, diagnosis, and management of polycystic ovary syndrome. Clin Epidemiol. 2014; 6: 1–13.

Chapter 2: The PCOS Spectrum: What PCOS Is and Is Not

1   El Hayek S et al. Poly cystic ovarian syndrome: an updated overview. Front Physiol. 2016; 7: 124.

2   Homburg R et al. Polycystic ovary syndrome: from gynaecological curiosity to multisystem endocrinopathy. Hum Reprod. 1996; 11: 29–39.

3   Kiddy DS et al. Improvement in endocrine and ovarian function during dietary treatment of obese women with polycystic ovary syndrome. Clin Endocrinol (Oxf). 1992; 36: 105–11.

4   Azziz R et al. Androgen excess in women: experience with over 1000 consecutive patients. J Clin Endocrinol Metab. 2004; 89(2): 453–62.

5   Eden J. The polycystic ovary syndrome presenting as resistant acne successfully treated with cyproterone acetate. Med J Aust. 1991; 155(10): 677–80.

6   Parker S. When missed periods are a metabolic problem. The Atlantic [Internet]. 2015 Jun 26. Available from: https://www.theatlantic.com/health/archive/2015/06/polycystic-ovary-syndrome-pcos/396116/. Accessed 2019 Aug 27.

7   Azziz R et al. The androgen excess and PCOS society criteria for the polycystic ovary syndrome: the complete task force report. Fertil Steril. 2009; 91(2): 456–88.

8   Mortensen M et al. Functional significance of polycystic-size ovaries in healthy adolescents. J Clin Endocrinol Metab. 2006; 91(10): 3786–90.

9   McCartney CR et al. Obesity and sex steroid changes across puberty: evidence for marked hyperandrogenemia in pre- and early pubertal obese girls. J Clin Endocrinol Metab. 2007; 92(2): 430–6.

Chapter 3: Who Gets PCOS?

1   Yildiz BO et al. Impact of obesity on the risk for polycystic ovary syndrome. J Clin Endocrinol Metab. 2008; 93: 162–68.

2   Vink JM et al. Heritability of polycystic ovary syndrome in a Dutch twin-family study. J Clin Endocrinol Metab. 2006; 91(6): 2100–4.

3   Legro RS et al. Evidence for a genetic basis for hyperandrogenemia in polycystic ovary syndrome. Proc Natl Acad Sci USA. 1998; 95(25): 14956–60.

4   Sam S et al. Evidence for metabolic and reproductive phenotypes in mothers of women with polycystic ovary syndrome. Proc Natl Acad Sci USA. 2006; 103(18): 7030–5.

5   Carmina E et al. Polycystic ovary syndrome (PCOS): arguably the most common endocrinopathy is associated with significant morbidity in women. J Clin Endocrinol Metab. 1999 June; 84(6): 1897–9.

6   Melo AS et al. Treatment of infertility in women with polycystic ovary syndrome: approach to clinical practice. Clinics (São Paulo). 2015 Nov; 70(11): 765–9.

7   Boyle J et al. Prevalence of infertility and use of fertility treatment in women with polycystic ovary syndrome: data from a large community-based cohort study. J Womens Health (Larchmt). 2015 Apr; 24(4): 299–307.

8   Azziz R et al. Health care-related economic burden of the polycystic ovary syndrome during the reproductive life span. J Clin Endocrinol Metab. 2005 Aug; 90(8): 4650–8. Some sources suggest these figures have remained stable over time; see: Al Bahar A. A look at the epidemiology of PCOS and economic cost to healthcare. PCOS Conference. 2015 Nov 16–18. [Internet] Available from: https://www.longdom.org/conference-abstracts-files/2161-1017.C1.011-020.pdf. Accessed 2019 Aug 27. The average cost of IVF treatments, however, has almost certainly increased since 2005.

9   Gray RH, Wu LY. Subfertility and risk of spontaneous abortion. Am J Public Health. 2000 Sep; 90(9): 1452–4.

10 Boomsma CM et al. A meta-analysis of pregnancy outcomes in women with polycystic ovary syndrome. Hum Reprod Update. 2006 Dec; 12(6): 673–83.

11 Norman JE et al. Progesterone for the prevention of preterm birth in twin pregnancy (STOPPIT): a randomised, double-blind, placebo-controlled study and meta-analysis. Lancet. 2009 Jun, 373(9680): 2034–40.

12 Boomsma CM et al. A meta-analysis of pregnancy outcomes in women with polycystic ovary syndrome. Hum Reprod Update. 2006 Dec; 12(6): 673–83.

13 Catalano PM et al. Gestational diabetes and insulin resistance: role in short- and long-term implications for mother and fetus. J Nutr. 2003 May; 133(5): 1674S–83S.

14 Silverman BL et al. Long-term effects of the intrauterine environment: The Northwestern University Diabetes in Pregnancy Center. Diabetes Care, suppl. Proceedings of the Fourth International Workshop-Conference, Alexandria. 1998 Aug; 21: B142–9. [Internet] Available from: https://search.proquest.com/openview/289566237c73175495f84f704ae9864d/. Accessed September 30, 2019.

15 Dahlgren E et al. Polycystic ovary syndrome and risk for myocardial infarction. Acta Obstet Gynecol Scand. 1992; 71: 599–604.

16 Solomon CG et al. Menstrual cycle irregularity and risk for future cardiovascular disease. J Clin Endocrinol Metab. 2002; 87: 2013–17.

17 Pierpoint T et al. Mortality of women with polycystic ovary syndrome at long term follow-up. J Clin Endocrinol Metab. 1998; 92: 240–5.

18 Wild RA et al. Assessment of cardiovascular risk and prevention of cardiovascular disease in women with the polycystic ovary syndrome: a consensus statement by the Androgen Excess and Polycystic Ovary Syndrome (AE-PCOS) Society. J Clin Endocrinol Metab. 2010; 95: 2038–49.

19 Ehrmann DA et al. Prevalence of impaired glucose tolerance and diabetes in women with polycystic ovary syndrome. Diabetes Care. 1999; 22(1): 141–6.

20 Kelley CE et al. Review of non-alcoholic fatty liver disease in women with polycystic ovary syndrome. World J Gastroenterol. 2014 Oct; 20(39): 14172–84.

21 Brown AJ et al. Polycystic ovary syndrome and severe non-alcoholic steatohepatitis: beneficial effect of modest weight loss and exercise on liver biopsy findings. Endocr Pract. 2005; 11: 319–24.

22 Rocha ALL et al. Non-alcoholic fatty liver disease in women with polycystic ovary syndrome: systematic review and meta-analysis. J Endocrinol Invest. 2017 Dec; 40(12): 1279–88.

23 Vassilatou E et al. Nonalcoholic fatty liver disease and polycystic ovary syndrome. World J Gastroenterol. 2014 July; 20(26): 8351–63.

24 Chrousos GP et al. Polycystic ovary syndrome is associated with obstructive sleep apnea and daytime sleepiness: role of insulin resistance. J Clin Endocrinol Metab. 2001; 86: 517–20.

25 Carmina E et al. Polycystic ovary syndrome (PCOS): arguably the most common endocrinopathy is associated with significant morbidity in women. J Clin Endocrinol Metab. 1999 Jun; 84(6): 1897–99.

26 Rasgon NL et al. Reproductive function and risk for PCOS in women treated for bipolar disorder. Bipolar Disord. 2005; 7(3): 246–259.

27 Clark AM et al. Weight loss results in significant improvement in pregnancy and ovulation rates in anovulatory obese women. Hum Reprod. 1995 Oct; 10(10): 2705–12.

28 Chittenden BG et al. Polycystic ovary syndrome and the risk of gynaecological cancer: a systematic review. Reprod Biomed Online. 2009; 19: 398–405.

29 Sandoiu A. Cancer: 40 percent of all cancers related to obesity, overweight. Medical News Today [Internet]. 2017 Oct 4. Available from: https://www.medicalnewstoday.com/articles/319639.php. Accessed 2019 Mar 27.

30 Peppard HR et al. Prevalence of polycystic ovary syndrome among premenopausal women with type 2 diabetes. Diabetes Care. 2001; 24: 1050–52.

31 Diamanti-Kandarakis E, Dunaif A. Insulin resistance and the polycystic ovary syndrome revisited: an update on mechanisms and implications. Endocrine Rev. 2012; 33: 981–1030.

32 Sawada M et al. Pregnancy complications and glucose intolerance in women with polycystic ovary syndrome. Endocr J. 2015; 62(11): 1017–23.

33 Leddy MA et al. The impact of maternal obesity on maternal and fetal health. Rev Obstet Gynecol. 2008; 1(4): 170–8.

34 Escobar-Morreale HF et al. High prevalence of the polycystic ovary syndrome and hirsutism in women with type 1 diabetes mellitus. J Clin Endocrinol Metab. 2000; 85(11): 4182–87.

35 Codner E et al. Diagnostic criteria for polycystic ovary syndrome and ovarian morphology in women with type 1 diabetes mellitus. J Clin Endrocrinol Metab. 2006; 91(6): 2250–56.

36 Reaven GM, Laws A, eds. Insulin resistance: The metabolic syndrome X. Totowa, NJ: Humana Press; 1999.

37 National Institutes of Health. Third Report of the National Cholesterol Education Program (NCEP) Expert Panel on Detection, Evaluation, and Treatment of High Blood Cholesterol in Adults (Adult Treatment Panel III). NIH Publication No. 02-5215. 2002 Sep. [Internet] Available from: https://www.nhlbi.nih.gov/files/docs/resources/heart/atp-3-cholesterol-full-report.pdf. Accessed 2019 Sep 30.

38 Gillings School of Global Public Health, University of North Carolina at Chapel Hill. Only 12 percent of American adults are metabolically healthy, Carolina study finds. 2018 Nov 28. [Internet] Available from: https://www.unc.edu/posts/2018/11/28/only-12-percent-of-american-adults-are-metabolically-healthy-carolina-study-finds/. Accessed 2019 Sep 30.

39 Azziz R et al. Health care-related economic burden of the polycystic ovary syndrome during the reproductive life span. J Clin Endocrinol Metab. 2005; 90: 4650–8. This figure seems to have remained stable over time; see: Al Bahar A. A look at the epidemiology of PCOS and economic cost to healthcare. PCOS Conference. 2015 Nov 16–18. [Internet] Available from: https://www.longdom.org/conference-abstracts-files/2161-1017.C1.011-020.pdf. Accessed 2019 Aug 27.

40 Azziz R et al. Health care-related economic burden of the polycystic ovary syndrome during the reproductive life span. J Clin Endocrinol Metab. 2005 Aug; 90(8): 4650–8.

41 Alvarez-Blasco F et al. Prevalence and characteristics of the polycystic ovary syndrome in overweight and obese women. Arch Intern Med. 2006; 166: 2081–6.

Chapter 4: What We Know about Obesity

1   Renew Bariatrics. Report: obesity rates by country—2017. 2017 Sep 23. [Internet] Available from: https://renewbariatrics.com/obesity-rank-by-countries/. Accessed 2019 Aug 27.

2   Redrawn from a figure at Lifestyleat.com. Body mass index to define your obesity level. [Internet] Available from: http://www.lifestyleat.com/body-mass-index-bmi-body-mass-index-to-define-your-obesity-level/. Accessed 2019 Aug 27.

3   US Department of Agriculture. A Brief History of USDA Food Guides. [Internet] Available from: https://www.choosemyplate.gov/eathealthy/brief-history-usda-food-guides. Accessed 2019 Sep 30.

4   Janney NW. The metabolic relationship of the proteins to glucose. J Biol Chem. 1915; 20: 321–50. See also: Hoover H et al. The metabolic response of subjects with type 2 diabetes to a high-protein, weight-maintenance diet. J Clin Endocrinol Metab. 2003 Aug; 88(8): 3577–83.

Chapter 5: Insulin: The Common Link between PCOS and Obesity

1   Diamanti-Kandarakis E. Role of obesity and adiposity in polycystic ovary syndrome. Int J Obes. 2007; 31: S8–13.

2   Figure uses data in Table 2 of Legro RS et al. Prevalence and predictors of risk for type 2 diabetes mellitus and impaired glucose tolerance in polycystic ovary syndrome: a prospective, controlled study in 254 affected women. J Clin Endocrinol Metab. 1999; 84(1): 165–69.

3   Borruel S et al. Global adiposity and thickness of intraperitoneal and mesenteric adipose tissue deposits are increased in women with polycystic ovary syndrome (PCOS). J Clin Endocrinol Metab. 2013; 98: 1254–63.

4   Alvarez-Blasco F et al. Prevalence and characteristics of the polycystic ovary syndrome in overweight and obese women. Arch Intern Med. 2006; 166: 2081–6.

5   Centers for Disease Control and Prevention. CDC grand rounds: childhood obesity in the United States. Morbidity and Mortality Weekly Report [Internet]. 2011 Jan 21. Available for free public use from: https://www.cdc.gov/mmwr/preview/mmwrhtml/mm6002a2.htm. Accessed 2019 Aug 27.

6   Silfen ME et al. Early endocrine, metabolic, and sonographic characteristics of polycystic ovary syndrome (PCOS): comparison between nonobese and obese adolescents. J Clin Endocrinol Metab. 2003; 88: 4682–8.

7   McCartney CR et al. The association of obesity and hyperandrogenemia during the pubertal transition in girls: obesity as a potential factor in the genesis of postpubertal hyperandrogenism. J Clin Endocrinol Metab. 2006; 91: 1714–22.

8   Escobar-Morreale HF et al. The polycystic ovary syndrome associated with morbid obesity may resolve after weight loss induced by bariatric surgery. J Clin Endocrinol Metab. 2005; 90: 6364–9.

9   Yildiz B et al. Impact of obesity on the risk for polycystic ovary syndrome. J Clin Endocrinol Metab. 2008; 93(1): 162–8.

Chapter 6: Insulin and Hyperandrogenism

1   Murray RD et al. Clinical presentation of PCOS following development of an insulinoma: case report. Hum Reprod. 2000 Jan; 15(1): 86–8.

2   Rosenfield RL, Ehrmann DA. The pathogenesis of polycystic ovary syndrome (PCOS): the hypothesis of PCOS as functional ovarian hyperandrogenism revisited. Endocr Rev. 2016 Oct; 37(5): 467–520.

3   Cedars MI et al. Long-term administration of gonadotropin-releasing hormone agonist and dexamethasone: assessment of the adrenal role in ovarian dysfunction. Fertil Steril. 1992; 57(3): 495–500.

4   Strain G et al. The relationship between serum levels of insulin and sex hormone-binding globulin in men: the effect of weight loss. J Clin Endocrinol Metab. 1994; 79(4): 1173–6.

5   Daka B et al. Inverse association between serum insulin and sex hormone-binding globulin in a population survey in Sweden. Endocr Connect. 2013 Mar; 2(1): 18–22.

6   Burghen GA et al. Correlation of hyperandrogenism with hyperinsulinism in polycystic ovarian disease. J Clin Endocrinol Metab. 1980; 50: 113–6.

7   Willis D et al. Modulation by insulin of follicle-stimulating hormone and luteinizing hormone actions in human granulosa cells of normal and polycystic ovaries. Clin Endocrinol Metab. 1996; 81: 302–9.

8   Micic D et al. Androgen levels during sequential insulin euglycemic clamp studies in patients with polycystic ovary disease. J Steroid Biochem. 1988; 31: 995–9.

9   Franks S et al. Insulin action in the normal and polycystic ovary. Endocrinol Metab Clin North Am. 1999; 28(2): 361–78.

10 Nestler JE et al. Suppression of serum insulin by diazoxide reduces serum testosterone levels in obese women with polycystic ovary syndrome. J Clin Endocrinol Metab. 1989; 68: 1027–32.

11 Geffner ME et al. Persistence of insulin resistance in polycystic ovarian disease after inhibition of ovarian steroid secretion. Fertil Steril. 1986; 45: 327–33.

12 Baillargeon JP et al. Commentary: polycystic ovary syndrome: a syndrome of ovarian hypersensitivity to insulin? J Clin Endocrinol Metab. 2006; 91(1): 22–4.

Chapter 7: Insulin, Polycystic Ovaries, and Anovulation

1   Dumesic DA et al. Ontogeny of the ovary in polycystic ovary syndrome. Fertil Steril. 2013 July; 100(1): 23–38.

2   Jonard S et al. The follicular excess in polycystic ovaries, due to intra-ovarian hyperandrogenism, may be the main culprit for the follicular arrest. Hum Reprod Update. 2004; 10(2): 107–17.

3   Webber LJ et al. Formation and early development of follicles in the polycystic ovary. Lancet. 2003; 362: 1017–21.

4   Redrawn from a figure in Franks S et al. Insulin action in the normal and polycystic ovary. Endocrinol Metab Clin North Am. 1999; 28(2): 361–78.

5   Franks S et al. Etiology of anovulation in polycystic ovary syndrome. Steroids. 1998; 63: 306–7.

6   Jonard S et al. The follicular excess in polycystic ovaries, due to intra-ovarian hyperandrogenism, may be the main culprit for the follicular arrest. Hum Reprod Update. 2004; 10(2): 107–17.

7   Kezele PR et al. Insulin but not insulin-like growth factor-1 promotes the primordial to primary follicle transition. Mol Cell Endocrinol. 2002; 192: 37–43.

8   Creanga AA et al. Use of metformin in polycystic ovary syndrome: a meta-analysis. Obstet Gynecol. 2008; 111(4): 959–68.

Chapter 8: Understanding the Roots of Insulin Resistance

1   Kahn CR et al. The syndromes of insulin resistance and acanthosis nigricans. Insulin-receptor disorders in man. N Engl J Med. 1976; 294: 739–45.

2   Musso C et al. Clinical course of genetic disease of the insulin receptor (Type A and Rabson-Mendenhall syndromes): a 30-year perspective. Medicine. 2004; 83(4): 209–22.

3   Burghen GA et al. Correlation of hyperandrogenism with hyperinsulinism in polycystic ovarian disease. J Clin Endocrinol Metab. 1980; 50: 113–6.

4   Dunaif A et al. Profound peripheral insulin resistance, independent of obesity, in polycystic ovary syndrome. Diabetes. 1989; 38: 1165–74.

5   Rosenfield RL et al. The pathogenesis of polycystic ovary syndrome (PCOS): the hypothesis of PCOS as functional ovarian hyperandrogenism revisited. Endocr Rev. 2016 Oct; 37(5): 467–520.

6   DeFronzo RA. Lilly lecture 1987. The triumvirate: beta-cell, muscle, liver. A collusion responsible for NIDDM. Diabetes. 1998; 37: 667–87.

Chapter 9: Medications and Surgery

1   de Melo, AS et al. Hormonal contraception in women with polycystic ovary syndrome: choices, challenges, and noncontraceptive benefits. Open Access J Contracept. 2017; 8: 13–23.

2   Bargiota A, Diamanti-Kandarakis E. The effects of old, new and emerging medicines on metabolic aberrations in PCOS. Ther Adv Endocrinol Metab. 2012 Feb; 3(1): 27–47.

3   Ibid.

4   McCartney CR, Marshall JC. Polycystic ovary syndrome. N Engl J Med. 2016; 375: 54–64.

5   Bargiota A, Diamanti-Kandarakis E. The effects of old, new and emerging medicines on metabolic aberrations in PCOS. Ther Adv Endocrinol Metab. 2012 Feb; 3(1): 27–47; Evans et al. Spironolactone in the treatment of idiopathic hirsutism and the polycystic ovary syndrome. J R Soc Med. 1986 Aug; 79(8): 451–3.

6   Agrawal NK. Management of hirsutism. Indian J Endocrinol Metab. 2013 Oct; 17(Suppl 1): S77–82.

7   Nestler JE, Jakubowicz DJ. Decreases in ovarian cytochrome P450c17α activity and serum free testosterone after reduction in insulin secretion in polycystic ovary syndrome. N Engl J Med. 1996; 335: 617–23.

8   Legro RS et al. Letrozole versus clomiphene for infertility in the polycystic ovary syndrome. N Engl J Med. 2014; 371: 119–29.

9   Morin-Papunen L et al. Metformin improves pregnancy and live-birth rates in women with polycystic ovary syndrome (PCOS): a multicenter, double-blind, placebo-controlled randomized trial. J Clin Endocrinol Metab. 2012 May; 97(5): 1492–500.

10 Vanky E et al. Metformin reduces pregnancy complications without affecting androgen levels in pregnant polycystic ovary syndrome women: results of a randomized study. Hum Reprod. 2004 Aug; 19(8): 1734–40.

11 Polycystic Ovary Syndrome Writing Committee. American Association of Clinical Endocrinologists position statement on metabolic and cardiovascular consequences of polycystic ovary syndrome. Endocr Pract. 2005; 11: 126–34.

12 Nasri H, Rafieian-Kopaei M. Metformin: current knowledge. J Res Med Sci. 2014 Jul; 19(7): 658–64.

13 Hjortrup A et al. Long-term clinical effects of ovarian wedge resection in polycystic ovarian syndrome. Acta Obstet Gynecol Scand. 1983; 62(1): 55–7.

14 Hendriks ML et al. Why does ovarian surgery in PCOS help? Insight into the endocrine implications of ovarian surgery for ovulation induction in polycystic ovary syndrome. Hum Reprod Update. 2007 May; 13(3): 249–64.

15 Mitra S et al. Laparoscopic ovarian drilling: an alternative but not the ultimate in the management of polycystic ovary syndrome. J Nat Sci Biol Med. 2015 Jan–Jun; 6(1): 40–8.

16 Katsikis M et al. Anovulation and ovulation induction. Hippokratia. 2006; 10(3): 120–12.

17 Legro RS et al. Letrozole versus clomiphene for infertility in the polycystic ovary syndrome. N Engl J Med. 2014; 371: 119–29.

18 Ibid.

19 Tarlatzis BC et al. Consensus on infertility treatment related to polycystic ovary syndrome. Fertil Steril. 2008; 89: 505–22.

20 Kansal Kalra S et al. Is the fertile window extended in women with polycystic ovary syndrome? Utilizing the Society for Assisted Reproductive Technology registry to assess the impact of reproductive aging on live-birth rate. Fertil Steril. 2013 Jul; 100(1): 208–13.

21 Lintsen AM et al. Effects of subfertility cause, smoking and body weight on the success rate of IVF. Hum Reprod. 2005 Jul; 20(7): 1867–75.

22 Azziz R et al. Health care-related economic burden of the polycystic ovary syndrome during the reproductive life span. J Clin Endocrinol Metab. 2005 Aug; 90(8): 4650–8.

23 Collins J. Cost-effectiveness of in vitro fertilization. Semin Reprod Med. 2001 Sep; 19(3): 279–89.

24 Legro RS et al. Letrozole versus clomiphene for infertility in the polycystic ovary syndrome. N Engl J Med. 2014; 371: 119–29.

25 Ibid.

26 Ibid.

Chapter 10: Low-Calorie Diets and Exercise

1 Moran LJ et al. Lifestyle changes in women with polycystic ovary syndrome. Cochrane Database Syst Rev. 2011 Feb; 2: CD007506.

2 Clark AM et al. Weight loss results in significant improvement in pregnancy and ovulation rates in anovulatory obese women. Hum Reprod. 1995 Oct; 10(10): 2705–12.

3 Clark AM et al. Weight loss in obese infertile women results in improvement in reproductive outcome for all forms of fertility treatment. Hum Reprod. 1998 Jun; 13(6): 1502–5.

4 Moran LJ et al. Dietary composition in the treatment of polycystic ovary syndrome: a systematic review to inform evidence-based guidelines. J Acad Nutr Diet. 2013 Apr; 113(4): 520–45; Douglas CC et al. Role of diet in the treatment of polycystic ovary syndrome. Fertil Steril. 2006 Mar; 85(3): 679–88.

5 Marsh K, Brand-Miller J. The optimal diet for women with polycystic ovary syndrome? B J Nutr. 2005 Aug; 94(2): 154–65.

6   Pfister K. The new faces of Coke. Medium [Internet]. 2015 Sep 8. Available from: https://medium.com/cokeleak/the-new-faces-of-coke-62314047160f. Accessed 2018 Dec 18.

7   Coca-Cola. Our commitment to transparency. 2017 Annual Review [Internet]. Available from: https://www.coca-colacompany.com/transparency/our-commitment-transparency. Accessed 2015 Apr 25.

8   O'Connor A. Coca-Cola funds scientists who shift blame away from bad diets. New York Times [Internet]. 2015 Aug 9. Available from: https://well.blogs.nytimes.com/2015/08/09/coca-cola-funds-scientists-who-shift-blame-for-obesity-away-from-bad-diets/?_r=0. Accessed 2019 Apr 25.

9   O'Connor A. Research group funded by Coca-Cola to disband. New York Times [Internet]. 2015 Dec 1. Available from: https://well.blogs.nytimes.com/2015/12/01/research-group-funded-by-coca-cola-to-disband/. Accessed 2019 Apr 25.

10 Howard BV et al. Low-fat dietary pattern and weight change over 7 years: The Women's Health Initiative Dietary Modification Trial. JAMA. 2006; 295: 39–49.

11 Redrawn from a figure in Howard BV et al. Ibid.

12 Tobey JA. The biology of human starvation. Am J Public Health Nations Health. 1951 Feb; 41(2): 236–7.

13 Hutchison SK et al. Effects of exercise on insulin resistance and body composition in overweight and obese women with and without polycystic ovary syndrome. J Clin Endocrinol Metab. 2011 Jan; 96(1): E48–56.

14 Giallauria F et al. Exercise training improves autonomic function and inflammatory pattern in women with polycystic ovary syndrome (PCOS). Clin Endocrinol (Oxf). 2008 Nov; 69(5): 792–8.

15 Harrison CL et al. Exercise therapy in polycystic ovary syndrome: a systematic review. Hum Reprod Update. 2011; 17(2): 171–83.

16 Lamb JD et al. Physical activity in women with polycystic ovary syndrome: prevalence, predictors, and positive health associations. Am J Obstet Gynecol. 2011; 204(4): 352.e1–6.

17 Ross R et al. Physical activity, total and regional obesity: dose-response considerations. Med Sci Sports Exerc. 2001; 33: S521–7.

18 Lee IM et al. Physical activity and weight gain prevention. JAMA. 2010; 303(12): 1173–9.

19 Clark AM et al. Weight loss results in significant improvement in pregnancy and ovulation rates in anovulatory obese women. Hum Reprod. 1995 Oct; 10(10): 2705–12.

20 Palomba S et al. Structured exercise training programme versus hypocaloric hyperproteic diet in obese polycystic ovary syndrome patients with anovulatory infertility: a 24-week pilot study. Hum Reprod. 2008 Mar; 23(3): 642–50.

21 Thomson RL et al. The effect of a hypocaloric diet with and without exercise training on body composition, cardiometabolic risk profile, and reproductive function in overweight and obese women with polycystic ovary syndrome. J Clin Endocrinol Metab. 2008 Sep; 93(9): 3373–80.

Chapter 11: The Optimal Diet for PCOS

1 Harcombe Z et al. Evidence from prospective cohort studies does not support current dietary fat guidelines: a systematic review and meta-analysis. Br J Sports Med. 2017 Dec; 51(24): 1743–9; Harcombe Z. Dietary fat guidelines have no evidence base: where next for public health nutritional advice? Br J Sports Med. 2017 May; 51(10): 769-74.

2 Howard BV et al. Low-fat dietary pattern and risk of cardiovascular disease: The Women's Health Initiative Randomized Controlled Dietary Modification Trial. JAMA. 2006 Feb; 295(6): 655–66.

3 Wang HS, Lin KL. Ketogenic diet: an early option for epilepsy treatment, instead of a last choice only. Biomed J. 2013 Jan-Feb; 36(1): 16–7; Groesbeck DK et al. Long-term use of the ketogenic diet in the treatment of epilepsy. Dev Med Child Neurol. 2006 Dec; 48(12): 978–81.

4 Popkin BM, Duffey KJ. Does hunger and satiety drive eating anymore? Am J Clin Nutr. 2010; 91: 1342–7.

5 Kahleova H et al. Meal frequency and timing are associated with changes in body mass index in Adventist Health Study 2. J Nutr. 2017 Sep; 147(9): 1722–8.

6 Gill S, Panda S. A smartphone app reveals erratic diurnal eating patterns in humans that can be modulated for health benefits. Clin Translat Rep. 2015 Nov; 22(5): 789–98.

7 Martin CK et al. Changes in food cravings during low-calorie and very-low-calorie diets. Obesity. 2006 Jan; 14(1): 115–21.

8 Kahathuduwa CN et al. Extended calorie restriction suppresses overall and specific food cravings: a systematic review and a meta-analysis. Obes Rev. 2017 Oct; 18(10): 1122–35.

9 Van Cauter E et al. Circadian modulation of glucose and insulin responses to meals: relationship to cortisol rhythm. Am J Physiol. 1992 Apr; 262(4 Pt 1): E467–76.

10 Scheer FA et al. The internal circadian clock increases hunger and appetite in the evening independent of food intake and other behaviors. Obesity. 2013 Mar; 21(3): 431–3.

11 Bo S et al. Is the timing of caloric intake associated with variation in diet-induced thermogenesis and in the metabolic pattern? A randomized cross-over study. Int J Obes (Lond). 2015 Dec; 39(12): 1689–95.

12 Being underweight is defined by Body Mass Index (BMI) under 18.5, but for a margin of safety I don't recommend that anybody with a BMI under 20 fast for extended periods.

13 Byrne NM et al. Intermittent energy restriction improves weight loss efficiency in obese men: the MATADOR study. Int J Obes (Lond). 2018 Feb; 42(2): 129–38.

14 Sutton EF et al. Early time-restricted feeding improves insulin sensitivity, blood pressure, and oxidative stress even without weight loss in men with prediabetes. Cell Metab. 2018 Jun; 27(6): 1212–21.e3.

15 Ibid.

Chapter 12: Practical Advice and Recipes for Women with PCOS

1 Sanger-Katz M. The decline of "big soda": the drop in soda consumption represents the single largest change in the American diet in the last decade. New York Times [Internet]. 2015 Oct 4. Available from: https://www.nytimes.com/2015/10/04/upshot/soda-industry-struggles-as-consumer-tastes-change.html. Accessed 2019 Aug 27.

2 Grassi D et al. Cocoa reduces blood pressure and insulin resistance and improves endothelium-dependent vasodilation in hypertensives. Hypertension. 2005 Aug; 46(2): 398–405.

3 Grassi D et al. Blood pressure is reduced and insulin sensitivity increased in glucose-intolerant, hypertensive subjects after 15 days of consuming high-polyphenol dark chocolate. J Nutr. 2008 Sep; 138(9): 1671–6.

4 Djoussé L et al. Chocolate consumption is inversely associated with prevalent coronary heart disease: the National Heart, Lung, and Blood Institute Family Heart Study. Clin Nutr. 2011 Apr; 30(2): 182–7.

5 MCT: medium-chain triglycerides. MCT oil is derived from coconut oil. It can be taken on its own or with food as an added source of fat and energy.

6 Chen IJ et al. Therapeutic effect of high-dose green tea extract on weight reduction: a randomized, double-blind, placebo-controlled clinical trial. Clin Nutr. 2016 Jun; 35(3): 592–9.

Recipe Index

General Index

....

Figures and tables indicated by page numbers in italics